D0862861

The Burning Truth

●

The Inspirational True Story of One Mother's Search
for the Answer to Her Teenage Son's Painful and
Highly Misunderstood Neurological Disorder,
Complex Regional Pain Syndrome (CRPS)

●

Wendy Weckstein

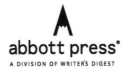

abbott press®
A DIVISION OF WRITER'S DIGEST

The Burning Truth

Abbott Press books may be ordered through booksellers or by contacting:

Abbott Press
1663 Liberty Drive
Bloomington, IN 47403
www.abbottpress.com
Phone: 1-866-697-5310

ISBN: 978-1-4582-0219-2 (sc)
ISBN: 978-1-4582-0221-5 (hc)
ISBN: 978-1-4582-0220-8 (e)

Library of Congress Control Number: 2012902691

Images on the book's cover were provided by Windborne Photographic Studios.

Printed in the United States of America

Abbott Press rev. date: 3/29/2012

"This book is the powerful account of the heroic struggle of one teen and his family against an unbearably painful and misunderstood illness. This book chronicles this brave young man's excruciating pain syndrome that developed following a tumble during horseplay with his brother, followed by a tireless search across the USA for help that lead to misunderstandings, dead ends, painful and frightening treatments, and, after extraordinary courage, to healing and recovery. This book is both an inspiring true story as well as an illuminating addition to the care of children and adolescents suffering from this poorly understood severe pain syndrome. I strongly recommend this book to both lay readers and professionals caring for children with chronic pain."

Kersti Bruining, M.D
Fellow of the American Academy of Neurology, Clinical Assistant Professor Department of Neurology and Ophthalmology, Michigan State University, Editorial Board of: *Continuum: Lifelong Learning in Neurology*®

"Wendy Weckstein's account of her son's illness is a heart-piercing story of suffering, honesty, courage, and determination. It is hard to think of another book populated by so many heroic people. Her story is not simply about a rare pain disorder. It should be read by every parent of any chronically ill child. But her story is larger than that. It's about the suffering that touches nearly every family in one form or another, and in that light, it should be read by us all."

Henry David Abraham, M.D.
Clinical professor in Psychiatry at Tufts University School of Medicine in Boston, Massachusetts, Co-recipient of the 1985 Nobel Peace Prize for his work with the International Physicians for the Prevention of Nuclear War, Author of "What's a Parent to Do? Straight Talk on Drugs and Alcohol," New Horizon Press.

"This is a compelling story of the saga of Devin's long journey through pain and the plight children in pain suffer from the illness and treatment in the medical community using the typical medical model. The disappointment, discouragement and harm that can come of these desperate attempts to control this desperate pain is gripping as we follow Devin until his ultimate cure. It is extremely hard to not directly attempt to treat the pain but force the body to cure itself through intense physical and occupational therapy along with psychological support. This is a condition that wreaks havoc on body, mind and soul but can be beat. We highly recommend *The Burning Truth* for all those who have such a child in their life and for all medical caregivers of children in chronic pain."

David D. Sherry, MD and Deborah Krepcio, CRNP
The Center for Amplified Musculoskeletal Pain Syndrome, the Children's Hospital of Philadelphia, Philadelphia, PA

"Hats off to a very resilient family and especially to Devin as he endured a torturous journey through an often uncomprehending and uncaring "health" system. Mrs. Weckstein's epilogue alone is well worth the price of this book."

Jim Broatch, MSW, Executive Director of the Reflex Sympathetic Dystrophy Syndrome Association, RSDSA

"*The Burning Truth* is an emotionally charged, first-hand account of one mother's fight to find healing for her son. Anyone with a child with CRPS or any chronic illness will find critically important encouragement, support and hope in these pages."

Meg Meeker, M.D., pediatrician and best-selling author

For all the children who suffer from Complex Regional Pain Syndrome (CRPS) and their families who support them.

Table of Contents

If children have the ability to ignore all odds and percentages, then maybe we can all learn from them. When you think about it, what other choice is there but to hope? We have two options, medically and emotionally: give up, or Fight Like Hell.

Lance Armstrong

Complex Regional Pain Syndrome (CRPS) – a Definition

Complex Regional Pain Syndrome (CRPS) is a rare neurological disorder characterized by intense and persistent burning, stabbing, or aching pain, extreme sensitivity to touch, swollen extremities that are exceedingly cold or hot, and often skin, nail, and bone changes. This debilitating disorder often confines its victims to wheelchairs, crutches, or even bed-rest if proper treatment isn't forthcoming.

CRPS often begins after a relatively minor injury to a limb or nerve. The pain becomes horrific and is often described as worse than the agony suffered by cancer victims or women going through labor and delivery. Its victims have described it as a burning fire that never goes out, a barbed wire wrapped around their skin, or a knife stabbing them repeatedly, 24 hours a day.

For reasons still not understood, CRPS develops after tissue damage from a trauma, such as a broken bone or injured nerve, when the nerves begin to misfire and continue to send pain signals to the brain even after the original injury or tissue damage has healed. As this occurs, the pain slowly starts to take on a life of its own. The nerves that carry the pain develop an overpowering and hyperactive circuit to the brain with no "off" button, like an engine revving out of control that cannot be stopped.

This constant pain is disproportionate to the original injury and often spreads. For example, even if the injury and pain are initially confined to just the foot, once CRPS develops, it can overtake the whole leg. Eventually, the pain becomes so bad that even the slightest touch makes its victim scream. Often, patients can't sleep, go to work or school, or take part in normal daily activities.

Few doctors have experience with CRPS. Consequently, this syndrome is highly misunderstood and extremely under-diagnosed. It typically takes over a year, sometimes much longer, to find the right doctor who can make the diagnosis and begin a treatment regimen. This situation is complicated by the fact that CRPS is also known as Reflex Sympathetic Dystrophy (RSD), Reflex Neurovascular Dystrophy (RND), or Amplified Musculoskeletal Pain Syndrome (AMPS), with doctors from different specialties utilizing different terminology as they treat the same disorder.

While they seek help, it is common for patients to be told, "It is all in your head" or "The pain is not real." The frustration these individuals and their loved ones feel is tremendous. The lucky ones eventually find a doctor who either has knowledge about this syndrome or is willing to find someone who does.

CRPS affects approximately 50,000 people a year in the United States. Although it can afflict both men and women, it is three times more common in women. CRPS can strike at any age, but is more prevalent in adults. Forty-two is the mean age of diagnosis, but CRPS has been diagnosed in children as young as three years of age. The number of cases among adolescents and young adults has not been estimated, but is reportedly on the rise.

Prologue

A Story Worth Telling

A mother's worst nightmare is watching her child suffer. Any mom can attest to the fact that she feels a strong instinctive drive to protect her child. When she can't, it hurts deep in her soul, penetrating well beyond what she ever thought possible; it is much worse than if she were going through the painful experience herself.

A severe injury or trauma to a child can lead to great despair, but when that child experiences unrelenting, debilitating, and agonizing pain day after day, it can literally rip you apart inside. As I discovered, a mother will do virtually anything to make the pain go away.

This is the true story of my son Devin who, at the age of 13 after a minor injury, developed a devastating neurological disorder known as Complex Regional Pain Syndrome (CRPS) and how he lived with constant unbearable pain for three years.

This is the story of our family's frustrating journey trying to make our son's pain go away and searching for the elusive cure, and it is the inspirational story of a boy who was dragged to hell but somehow summoned up the courage, strength, and determination to find his way back without losing himself along the way.

This is also the story of the many difficult and disturbing truths I was forced to confront as Devin's devastating condition slowly took over our lives. The most profound and recurrent awakening centered around vast flaws within our modern-day medical system, especially when it comes to the diagnosis and treatment of pain.

To my surprise, I learned that even the most reputable of physicians, instead of trusting their patients, are prone to labeling

1

inconclusive and hard-to-diagnose pain as psychosomatic. This maddening reality, along with the rarity of CRPS, caused us to flounder for many months.

At times, my personal anguish was nearly overwhelming and I often felt paralyzed as I watched my son's condition deteriorate. Needing to find the answer and having no other alternative, I channeled my distress into sheer determination as I accompanied Devin through what seemed to be never-ending airport corridors around the country in search of a doctor who would not only understand what was wrong with him but would also believe in him.

Ultimately, this book chronicles the life lessons I was forced to learn as I dealt with my on-going private feelings of despair and helplessness even while I remained determinedly optimistic in front of Devin.

Our son endured numerous painful surgical procedures, disabling medications, controversial and dangerous treatments, and weeks in intensive care units as we desperately attempted to control and end his suffering. As I sat by his side, the importance of trusting my instincts as a mother and being a strong advocate for him became crystal clear. Of necessity, I learned the fine art of navigating through both the medical system and the school system as I addressed Devin's unexpected and previously nonexistent special needs.

Teachers and administrators had to be creative and flexible and required continuous guidance to deal effectively and fairly with the sudden onset of Devin's debilitating physical condition and the challenging cognitive and visual deficits he experienced as a result of the strong pain medications he took.

Inevitably, conflicts arose that had to be addressed. The only way I could manage this was by staying confident and never hesitating when it came to trusting my instincts. Early on, I committed one big error in this regard, but I learned from this mistake and made sure it didn't happen again.

A lesson I wish I could have skipped was learning firsthand

about the inconsistencies inherent in the new Michigan Medical Marijuana law. Unfortunately, allowing Devin to use medical marijuana for a brief time was unavoidable. This unsettling four-month period revealed a world of false motives, legal discrepancies, and an inexcusable lack of professionalism. Although I saw the miraculous effect cannabis can have on the reduction of pain, I also witnessed the rather disconcerting realities surrounding medical marijuana and the inevitable psychological dependency that comes from its use.

By remaining hopeful and optimistic, even when it seemed as if all hope was gone, we were able to avoid relying on marijuana as a palliative solution for Devin and instead continued our search for the permanent answer to his painful condition.

It was our hope, along with our unshakeable belief that living with this type of pain for the rest of his life could not and would not be our child's destiny, that provided Devin with the courage and strength to keep going during the most difficult times. He had trust and confidence in us, and if we remained hopeful, so did he.

The fact is, these three years were truly horrific, a nightmare from which I am only recently being awakened. Through all the craziness I experienced and the trauma Devin endured, I kept a journal. I was frequently alone with Devin for lengthy periods in hospitals and doctors' offices throughout the country while he received aggressive and at times dangerous medical treatments. At these times, my husband and other two children did their best to proceed with life as usual at home. Sander, a child psychiatrist, accompanied us to many in-state doctors' appointments, but of necessity he also continued working. Ethan and Taylor, thankfully, had school, friends, and sports to focus on.

Devin's life and my life turned completely upside down. I am a physical therapist and had just started my own business as a fitness and wellness consultant for women when Devin's injury occurred. My schedule was full yet flexible, so for a short period of time I was able to continue seeing my clients. Within a couple of months of his injury, Devin's pain became unbearable and his needs all-consuming. We began our travels searching for an answer, and I put my business on hold.

Soon, our bright, active, and social young son could no longer take part in any of the normal activities of a typical 13-year-old boy. He could not play sports, go on social outings with his friends, join family activities, or regularly attend or succeed in school. Instead, his life was controlled by his pain.

In many respects, this was a very lonely and frightening time, and nightly phone calls home during the periods we were away could only provide so much comfort. Sander and I always made treatment decisions together, and I received regular supportive phone calls from wonderful friends, but I was often on my own to comfort and care for Devin as the treatments themselves progressed. Missing Sander, Ethan, and Taylor, worried about them, and increasingly afraid for Devin, I needed a way to vent at any time of the day or night without feeling like a burden.

My journal became the tireless friend I so badly needed. Recapping each experience in writing helped me process what was happening, as if I were pricking myself to see if I were awake or just in a really bad dream.

At times, I found that my journal became almost a living person. Sometimes all I wanted to do was retreat to a corner and write. At the worst of times, writing in my journal was the one thing that could center me and help me make sense of the chaos all around me.

Chaos? It's not too strong a word. Between Devin's pain and the extremes we went to trying to control and cure it, a somewhat controlled chaos became routine for everyone in our family. I suspect many readers will be alarmed and perhaps even appalled by some of the decisions we made in the course of trying to treat Devin's pain. All I ask is that readers try to put themselves in our shoes. I would not wish this experience on my worst enemy, and I am profoundly grateful we survived it.

Revising my personal journal into a book meant for public

consumption has been cathartic. I hope that by telling Devin's complicated story, others can avoid some of the mistakes and poor choices we made. I hope that by sharing this occasionally unbelievable and intrinsically fascinating journey, other families who have a child afflicted with CRPS will find it a bit easier to navigate through the complicated morass of this highly misunderstood syndrome and its accompanying world of pain.

Above all, I hope this story will inspire others to never give up hope while looking for the answer to their illness, or to any personal life crisis, and I hope it helps them find the determination and courage to triumph over it once they do.

Chapter 1

An Innocent-Looking Tumble,
and the Nightmare Begins

August 30, 2009

Devin and I are finally on our way to the Children's Hospital of Philadelphia. Staring out the airplane window at the beautiful sky, I wonder... am I about to wake up from this nightmare? Is my fifteen year old son about to have his life back?

Devin is sleeping peacefully on my shoulder and I can't help hold back my tears; will he actually wake up in a few short weeks knowing what it's like to live again without pain? I smile as I think about this amazing vision but my insides are still tight with anxiety. Devin has been through so much; the worst kind of torture any teenager could imagine since he was just 13. I get so frustrated when I think that Dr. Sherry's program in Philadelphia had been there all along and we just couldn't find it. Two bright, medically educated parents, yet we somehow couldn't find the one program that may finally be the answer!

It sickens me to think about all that Devin's endured; 15 doctors, 14 medication trials, 12 surgical procedures, 4 horrible weeks in intensive care units where we had him receive risky treatments like ketamine infusions...all because he was suffering and we didn't know what the hell to do! The amount of money wasted by us and our insurance company as he received one failed treatment after another was obscene.

I can't believe we were moments away from sending him to Germany to put him in a ketamine coma! Devin's pain was so unbearable - but a coma in another country - for the love of god, what were we thinking?

Who knew that medical marijuana would become his only reliable source of relief? What an outrageous experience that turned out to be. All I can say is, I'm glad those days are over!

What is totally amazing is that Devin is still on track with school. Thank goodness for some really great teachers, but I sure hope that I never come that close again to taking the school to hearing because of their insensitivity to special needs!

I think back at how truly horrific this has been for Devin - for our whole family - all because of a minor injury 2 years ago, that really should have been No Big Deal ...

September 15, 2007, was the night of the big soccer game between the northern Michigan small-town rivals Central High School and West Senior High School. Devin, who had just begun the eighth grade, had been invited to attend the game with his big brother Ethan, a junior at Central. What began as a kind act of brotherly love turned into the catalyst that changed Devin's life, all our lives, in ways we never could have imagined.

Ethan was Central High School's biggest fan. Inevitably dressed in black and gold face paint and matching wacky clothes, Ethan was that noisy, noticeable student in the fan section leading the other students in loud chants and cheers. His lack of inhibition and enthusiasm probably made him one of the best super fans the school has ever seen!

I often heard from friends who regularly attended these high school sporting events that they were more entertained by my son's high energy theatrics up in the bleachers than by the gripping game being played on the field below.

Devin, being an easygoing low-key sort of guy, was in great awe of his big brother's larger-than-life personality. Both he and his little sister Taylor, with her freckled face and long red curly hair, found their confident, crazy, outgoing older brother hysterical and entertaining.

Devin had been hoping to see his brother in action at one of these games and was thrilled by the invitation. He was in the middle of a marathon piano practicing session after school when, at the last minute, Ethan asked if he wanted to go.

He dropped his piano books in an instant and ran into the kitchen, asking, "Mom, can I please go to the soccer game with Ethan tonight?"

I was preparing dinner and hesitated. It was a school night after all, but that was more of an excuse than anything. The fact was, sending him off with Ethan and his big sixteen-year-old friends and their new sixteen-year-old driver's licenses would take some getting used to.

But, the evenings were still warm and summer-like and the pressures of school had not yet begun. The game would be over before dark, I reasoned. Besides, it warmed my heart that Ethan wanted to spend time with his little brother and that he'd asked him to join him at the big game.

"Sure," I said with a smile on my face. "Have a good time."

"Ethan," I yelled into the other room, "be sure to bring Devin home right after the game. Don't forget you both have school tomorrow!"

"Okay, no problem," said Ethan, as he ran into the kitchen and gave me a big kiss on the cheek. "We've got to go. The game starts in a few minutes and my friends are waiting outside."

"Thanks, Mom. I'll see you later!" Devin ran after his brother out the door.

* * *

Later that evening at the jam-packed field, Devin innocently hopped onto Ethan's shoulders as they both began cheering for the home team. It was a close match with the score tied at 2-2, and the students were exceptionally rowdy. Unfortunately, at a high point in the game, when a goal was scored and the fans were going wild, Devin lost his balance and tumbled off his brother's shoulders onto the hard-packed soil, landing flat on his tailbone.

After several moments, a bit stunned from the fall, Devin gradually rose from the ground. Finding that he couldn't sit on his sore behind, he spent the remainder of the game leaning against the bleachers. He wasn't about to tell his cool older brother, who had invited him to tag along, that he was hurting and wanted to go home. No, he would stick it out no matter how uncomfortable he was. He refused to be the party pooper, so instead of telling Ethan the truth when asked if he was okay, Devin yelled above the noisy crowd and told him he was just fine.

When the boys got home a couple of hours later, Ethan came bounding through the front door, still unaware of how much Devin was hurting. He told us about the great game while Devin slowly limped in behind.

As Devin told us about his fall, he chuckled, dismissing his pain as a funny outcome of making the wrong choice to cheer for the team while perched on his brother's shoulders.

We assured him he probably just had a nasty bruise around his tailbone that would most likely get better over the next few days. While we talked to him about the importance of icing the painful area and perhaps taking it easy during the upcoming week, Devin's gaze shifted towards the living room at his beloved baby grand.

"In the meantime," I told him with a smile, "a nice soft pillow for your piano bench might be a good idea."

Devin had developed a great passion for music at a young age and had started playing the piano when he was just three years old. He practiced and entertained us with classical and jazz pieces for hours each day, and until his tailbone was less tender, sitting on that hard wooden surface was surely going to be a problem.

Nothing pointed to a serious injury, but for some reason I had a sinking feeling inside as I watched Devin slowly walk to his room that night before bed. I could see that each step he took caused him pain, and I agreed with Sander that we should take him in for an x-ray if he was still limping in a couple of days.

Maybe it was just my motherly instinct, but I distinctly remember how truly uncomfortable I felt that evening. I hated seeing any of my children in pain. It tore me apart inside, and I always wished I could assume their suffering for them.

Little did I know this feeling would consume every ounce of my being for the next three years.

*   *   *

It quickly became evident that what seemed to be a very soar tailbone was something a bit more serious. Two days after his fall, Devin began to complain of tremendous burning pain traveling down his right leg. He could barely put weight on it, and soon he even began having a hard time lifting his right foot up to take a step.

The physical therapist in me roared to life. A quick assessment revealed that in addition to his extremely soar behind, Devin had significant weakness and pain down his right leg following a specific nerve pattern.

Instantly, that sinking feeling returned. This meant there was probably some degree of nerve damage from the impact of the fall. I was now officially worried, for I knew that nerve damage could be serious and even a mild case could take a long time to heal.

That weekend, Sander and I decided to take our still sore son to see my father, a family practitioner in a small town nearby. A good old-fashioned family doctor, I knew I could count on him to further assess Devin and give us some good advice.

He confirmed that Devin's symptoms pointed to some degree of nerve damage, but because this wasn't his area of expertise, he decided to refer us to a local specialist for a more thorough evaluation. He also made arrangements for Devin to receive an MRI the next day so we could get a better look at his spinal column.

By Tuesday, the results of Devin's MRI were back. The images were normal and revealed no damage to the nerves within his spine. This was good news, but we still kept our appointment with the specialist my father had recommended, a physical medicine and rehabilitation doctor in our hometown of Traverse City. Maybe he could explain why, nearly two weeks after his injury, Devin's pain wasn't improving.

*   *   *

Due to a recent cancellation, we were thankful to get an appointment with this physician for the following week. Unfortunately, this is where our gratitude ended. Upon meeting with the doctor, after waiting an agonizing hour and a half past our appointment time, he quickly introduced himself, asked Devin a few brief questions, and then began to perform a strength test on his right leg.

Within moments I began to feel uneasy. Having sat in the waiting room for such an extended length of time, I was amazed when the doctor rushed through Devin's history. I was at least expecting an ample amount of time to visit with him as a reward for our patience. Obviously this was not going to be the case.

I became even more uncomfortable as I watched him perform his exam. As a physical therapist, manual muscle testing is my bread and butter, and his technique was incorrect. By improperly assessing Devin's strength, he was seeing inconsistencies that could make it easy for him to conclude that Devin was faking his strength test. I bit my lip and decided to wait until the end of the visit to discuss this with him.

To my surprise, I didn't have the opportunity. The visit lasted at most 15 minutes, with no time to hear about the details of Devin's injury or his pain. The doctor told us Devin most likely had a nerve root contusion or bruise from the fall and that it would heal in eight to ten weeks. He prescribed a pain medication called Neurontin, abruptly ended the appointment, and scurried off to see his next patient.

Although the nerve root contusion was probably a good guess as to why Devin was experiencing such pain, especially since his MRI was normal, I left the office uncomfortable with both the evaluation and the way the appointment had concluded. The doctor had shown little respect for Devin, lacked competence in an important skill that is crucial for specialists in his field, and was quick to make judgments based on inaccurate information. It was difficult to accept this, but since I thought the diagnosis was probably correct and I knew he was a smart and respected doctor, I took a "wait and see" approach.

* * *

During the next few days, I continued to have a twinge of concern that something more was going on, but by now the Neurontin had begun to relieve Devin's pain, so I decided to let time take its course. What was the point, I told myself, in confronting the specialist? What good would it do?

I felt horrible that Devin would miss tennis, his favorite sport, for the next two or three months while he healed, but that couldn't be helped. In the meantime, I would have him do some gentle exercises at home so that he could keep that leg as strong as possible while we waited for his nerve root to heal. He still had to take it easy for a while until the inflammation went down, but the specialist had commented that complete rest was out of the question, and I agreed. This would only have encouraged Devin to avoid using his painful leg altogether. If possible, we needed him to continue using his right leg to keep it from getting weaker or developing the plethora of other problems that could occur from lack of use.

However, in spite of my best efforts, Devin's leg seemed to be getting weaker and weaker right before my eyes. The gentle exercises I had him doing just weren't enough. To make matters worse, he was now favoring his right leg all the time by limping, even hopping from one room of the house to another in order to avoid the terrific pain that came from putting weight on it.

So, with his physician's approval, I decided to increase Devin's exercise program. His injury was now more chronic in nature, and his doctor confirmed there was less worry about aggravating the nerve root.

The new program was more intense and took Devin a good 45 minutes to complete each day. It included riding the stationary bike, swimming at the local pool, and doing a whole series of leg exercises with stretch bands and light weights. Progress was slow to nonexistent, but Devin took his pain medicine and conscientiously followed his exercise program each day without complaint.

*   *   *

Throughout this period, life more or less went on as usual for the rest of the family. Sander's practice kept him busy, and Ethan was deeply involved in the high school musical, the varsity tennis team, his friends, his girlfriend, and the heavy academic requirements of his junior year.

Taylor, a fourth grader, was in the midst of soccer season, playing loads of tennis herself, and hanging out with friends. Our little Leonardo De Vinci also liked to spend countless hours sketching the human form in black and white and creating invention after invention in her special little notebook.

I kept a careful eye on Devin and his therapy while juggling our home, acting as glorified chauffeur for numerous hectic schedules, and working part-time in my new business. Fall in the northern Michigan resort community of Traverse City is lovely, and in spite of our busy lives, we all enjoyed the beauty of the twin bays that surround the peninsula we live on.

We were taken aback when, about six weeks after his original injury, Devin's pain began to worsen. He could bear even less weight on his leg now, and it was red and felt ice cold most of the time.

I was confused. Devin's pain should have been going away, his leg getting stronger. What was going on here? Why was his condition getting worse instead of better? Was this normal for a simple nerve root injury? Was there more nerve damage than we'd originally thought?

I began to wonder if we should have done an electromyography (EMG) or nerve conduction test.

For continuity's sake and because this was his specialty, we returned to the same doctor.

*   *   *

After another hour-long wait, the physician entered the room, said a quick "hello," and repeated the same improperly performed manual muscle assessment.

In hindsight, I'm not sure what I was expecting. All I know is that I was beginning to question my decision to return to his office. Puzzled by my own judgment, I sat in the chair opposite Devin as he lay on the exam table waiting for the EMG, a procedure that involved inserting numerous needles into his already painful and highly sensitive right leg muscles to measure electrical activity.

Not being the most insightful of physicians, the specialist abruptly began the test without telling Devin how painful it would be. Devin is a tough kid, but you could see from his grimacing face that he was shocked and unprepared for this degree of pain.

Puncturing his leg one needle at a time, I watched as the doctor silently twisted and maneuvered each needle deep within the muscles of Devin's right leg, offering no comforting small talk or even a clear explanation as to what he was doing. Fifteen minutes later, after he withdrew the last probe, the doctor read the results and concluded that the EMG was normal. This meant there was no sign of severe nerve damage and I took a deep breath of relief, but this good news only confused me further. I asked if the nerve root contusion itself could still be responsible for the weakness and worsening pain Devin was experiencing.

At this, the doctor pulled me aside and confirmed the premonition I'd had at our first appointment. Privately, he told me that although he believed Devin had some pain, he thought he was faking his weakness.

Knowing his assessment of Devin's strength was based on the inaccurate manual muscle test he'd now improperly performed *twice*, I carefully tried to explain what had gone wrong in his testing and why his assessment was inaccurate. I wasn't angry or rude, merely intent on getting to the bottom of why Devin was so weak and continuing to feel such pain.

In response, the doctor told me the visit was over. After quickly scribbling out a prescription increasing the dose of Devin's pain medication, he unceremoniously left the room.

I cannot describe my astonishment at this development. My 13-year-old son, who had never seen a diagram on nerve innervations, was able to confabulate to the last detail weakness in the fourth and fifth lumbar nerve down his right leg? (This, by the way, had taken me a number of late nights in the library to memorize while studying neurology back in college.) I figured I either had a prodigy who must promptly become a neurologist when he grew up, or this doctor was inept. Whether he didn't believe Devin or simply didn't know why Devin's pain was worse, we had a problem.

Forget this doctor's inaccurate perception of Devin's weakness; forget his insensitivity and lack of bedside manner. He was still a physician in a specialty that should be able to explain and treat this problem. Despite Devin's exercise program at home, his pain was worsening. Even more maddening, it was spreading – his entire leg had become so hypersensitive that if someone accidentally kicked, bumped, or even lightly rubbed up against it, his pain skyrocketed out of control.

Obviously, we needed a new physician. We needed someone who would listen closely to Devin's complaints and history. We needed someone who would trust Devin and believe in him. This doctor had made inaccurate judgments based on rushing and poor testing techniques; Devin had not and would not receive proper treatment from him. We needed a doctor who, if he didn't understand what was going on, would help us find the right specialist who could help our son.

Chapter 2

Two Steps Backward,
One Step Forward Towards a Diagnosis

December 8, 2007

I don't know what to do. Devin is calling me almost every day telling me he's in too much pain to stay at school. He's miserable! I've never seen him like this before. It's really starting to scare me. Nobody can go anywhere near his leg. If someone rubs against it, he screams and it sets off a terrible reaction where his pain flies off the chart!

And now he's failing his classes. That's the least of my concerns, but it's like this nightmare keeps getting worse. On his heavy pain medicine, he's falling asleep in class, he can't concentrate, and to top it off he can't read anymore because his vision is so blurry. Truthfully, in this debilitated state he can barely function at school. I'm meeting with all of his teachers and the principal tomorrow, but I really don't know what to tell them.

Devin's pain has completely consumed me. It's unbearable for me to keep watching him suffer like this! Right now though, I have to organize my thoughts, figure out a way to help these teachers work with Devin in this condition, and somehow get this kid to pass the 8th grade.

Grim, disappointed, and determined, we contacted a pediatric orthopedic doctor friend of ours from Grand Rapids, Michigan. He listened to our plight and agreed to get Devin on his busy schedule as soon as possible.

However, by the time Dr. Michael Forness was able to see Devin two weeks later, our son was experiencing a whole new set of problems. The higher dose of Neurontin he had begun taking kept his pain under control a bit better, but it also caused him to be extremely tired, dizzy, and uncoordinated. His thinking became fuzzy, and he developed such blurry vision that he could no longer read most texts and homework sheets.

Within a few short weeks, our straight A student in the district's talented and gifted program was struggling to pass his classes. He hobbled along at such a slow pace that he could no longer get to class on time, and on more than one occasion, groggy from the medicine, he fell asleep during class. Even when he could keep his eyes open, he had a hard time understanding the material. He was either in too much pain to concentrate or too foggy to understand what he was being taught.

I spent an inordinate amount of time explaining his condition to his teachers and helping them come up with ideas to get around his challenges. I suggested blowing up his assignments or using books on tape and even skipping assignments that weren't absolutely necessary. I requested a pass so he could be late to his classes. Adding insult to injury, I also asked that he be excused from his classes 10 minutes early so he could shuffle to his locker without encountering the otherwise heavy traffic of normal dismissal time.

Much to the school administrator's dismay, I wouldn't allow him to use crutches or a wheelchair, knowing such devices would only hasten the weakening of his leg. I also knew that if he got into a wheelchair and no longer had to put weight on that painful leg, he would never want to get out.

Devin's teachers were understanding and did their best, but inevitably they would forget our discussions and become frustrated. I would patiently set up meetings and kindly remind them again and again what Devin was going through, but sometimes I felt like I was getting nowhere. After all, how much can a teacher take when, in addition to being absent from school, a student comes to class late, falls asleep during lectures, and doesn't follow through with assignments?

On the outside, I remained optimistic and told his teachers we would soon learn what was causing this pain, but inside, my feelings of hopelessness were growing. Devin's pain was unbearable and seemed to be getting worse with each day, and the medicine, though only partially controlling it, was rendering him almost completely dysfunctional.

The severity of Devin's condition was highlighted one day at school in mid-November when a chair toppled onto his right foot during class as a student rocked back and forth in his seat. My mild-mannered, well-behaved, 13-year-old son shocked his teacher and classmates during a history lecture with a deafening and extremely drawn out, "F…U…C…K!" that resonated throughout the hallways and instantly brought his class to silence and him to his knees.

As horrified as I was to hear that Devin had bellowed out this obscenity in the middle of social studies class, I knew this wasn't his typical response. Devin usually kept his pain quietly to himself and tried hard not to draw attention or make a scene. Sometimes he literally came home with teeth marks on his forearm, which he'd bitten in order to keep from screaming out loud when his leg was bumped.

For the most part, his teachers and most kids, minus his closest friends, never knew when his pain was too much to bear. Nonetheless, as the weeks went by, he quietly and increasingly went to the office, called me, and told me he couldn't make it through the day.

I would stop whatever I was doing, drive to school, and take him home. Invariably, I found my son barely able to talk. He was never dramatic, crying, screaming, or ranting. Instead, he withdrew into himself, privately enduring his personal agony.

His silence and quiet resolve were the worst part. It was torture to watch him suffer this way.

We were thankful Devin had distractions during this very difficult period. His wonderful group of friends and his passion for the piano could almost always bring a smile to his face. At the time, Devin was taking jazz and classical piano lessons in the hopes of attending Interlochen Arts Academy, a renowned performing arts high school. This meant about two hours of practice each evening.

In and of itself this demanding practice schedule wasn't a problem – Devin hadn't gone one day without playing the piano since he'd started this instrument at age three – but combined with swimming after school, home exercises, doctor's appointments, the all-consuming homework necessary to stay caught up with his classmates, and the debilitating side effects of his medication, Devin was more than a bit overwhelmed.

Something had to give, and I worked with Devin and his teachers to help take off as much pressure as possible while we desperately tried to figure out what was wrong. Fortunately, keeping Devin focused and structured with schoolwork, exercises, and piano was generally easy, thanks to his easygoing nature. He was extremely motivated to keep up with his classmates, and we were impressed by his willingness to exercise each day if this would help make his pain go away.

Don't get me wrong; there certainly were many times when his pain was simply crushing, usually after a bump or minor injury. On these days, Devin wouldn't even sit down at the piano. Prior to his injury, it was rare for a single evening to pass without "Afternoon in Paris" or a Chopin prelude loudly playing in the background while I prepared dinner. When Devin lay on the couch, refused to go near his most prized possession, and communicated with one-syllable grunts, we knew his pain was unbearable.

*   *   *

Our entire family was tremendously relieved when the day came to drive Devin to Grand Rapids. Dr. Forness performed an excellent evaluation and immediately agreed with the nerve-related weakness. He also spent almost an hour assessing everything possible orthopedic and neurological. He took sacral x-rays and had us repeat a lumbosacral MRI just in case anything had changed. Most importantly, he spent plenty of time listening to Devin and trying to make sense of the injury.

Although the repeat MRI had to wait until the next day, the sacral x-rays were taken during that visit and analyzed immediately. Since all the other testing had come back normal, I wasn't surprised to learn the x-rays showed no abnormality.

Increasingly frustrated, I expressed to Dr. Forness my concern that we couldn't seem to pinpoint what was making Devin's condition worse.

Also puzzled, Dr. Forness mentioned the possibility that Devin might have a neurological disorder known as Reflex Sympathetic Dystrophy (RSD), also called Complex Regional Pain Syndrome, or CRPS for short. He explained that with an injury like a nerve root contusion, the nervous systems in patients with CRPS will continue to fire aggressive and constant pain signals to the brain, and although the nerve root may continue to get better, the pain will systematically get worse and sometimes take on a life of its own.

CRPS seemed to fit the bill, but Dr. Forness admitted he had little experience with this disorder. He thought a referral to the pain clinic associated with his hospital made the most sense. The clinic treated this disorder and could possibly help confirm the diagnosis. It could also provide an out-patient surgical spinal procedure known as a sympathetic block that would hopefully help Devin's pain.

Devin and I followed Dr. Forness' advice. Later that week, we drove to this pain clinic, two hours from home, where Devin saw a wonderful physician who concurred with the diagnosis of CRPS and administered the first of three separate sympathetic spinal blocks. This was an invasive surgical procedure and a much bigger deal than either of us had envisioned, but Devin was ready and extremely hopeful that it would help with his pain.

During each visit, Devin was taken into surgery and two

impressively long needles were inserted next to his spinal cord. The first injected a dye for the purpose of viewing the targeted area on an overhead x-ray machine, and the second transferred analgesics and other medications to the injured nerve root area.

Devin received a sympathetic spinal block three weeks in a row, but this procedure provided no reprieve from the pain.

* * *

Meanwhile, the torture of watching my son in pain 24 hours a day, knowing there was no way I could help him, was indescribable. I was simultaneously paralyzed by the sadness of this reality and frantically searching for an answer. I was also caught up in the day-to-day routine of caring for a chronically ill child without dropping the ball on the other responsibilities that came with running a busy family of five. Between keeping up with Devin's educational, physical, and medical needs, trying to somehow keep my business afloat, and tending to the usual bills, laundry, cleaning, shopping, meals, social obligations, after-school activities, field trips, college prep requirements, and dentist, doctor, and orthodontist appointments, I often felt like I was barely managing.

"I'm organized and strong, and I am not going to have the rest of my family suffer," I told myself. "I can do this!"

I kept it together on the outside, but inside I was starting to crack. Devin's pain was consuming our whole house, and it was becoming hard to disguise this reality. With the help of my wonderful husband and really no other choice, I soldiered on with the two main goals of keeping our family functioning and finding the answer to Devin's pain.

Sander and I began devouring everything we could find about CRPS on the internet. We greatly appreciated Dr. Forness pointing us in the right direction, and based on everything we could find, we agreed with his diagnosis. We wanted to learn as much as we could about this terrible disease and every possible treatment available.

Devin's pain was taking over his life, and we needed an answer soon.

In spite of the medicine he was taking, his pain hovered at a 7 ½ out of 10 on the pain scale universally used to assess pain. His nights had become miserable and sleep deprivation was taking its toll. His sensitivity to touch was worsening and the slightest contact on that leg set him off terribly. He could barely walk, and couldn't participate in any normal physical activities for a teenager his age. He certainly couldn't play tennis, which meant his dream of playing on the high school team the following fall was quickly slipping away.

Halfway through his eighth grade year, four and a half months after his original injury, we were watching Devin become ever more dysfunctional while suffering increasing pain each day. Our best efforts to help him had been unproductive, and Sander and I were becoming increasingly scared, with absolutely no idea of where to turn next.

Chapter 3

High Hopes and a Big Mistake

January 11, 2008

Keeping a journal has been good for me. It seems to help me process what's going on, but more importantly I'm really starting to see how crucial it is that I document everything that's happening with Devin's care. He's already had so many tests, seen so many doctors, and had so many procedures, that I think it will help us keep track of it all.

It's now 3:00 in the morning and I should really go to sleep, but every time I try I just keep tossing and turning. I tried to read, but I can't seem to concentrate. My mind is racing and tonight I feel sick to my stomach.

Watching Devin live with this kind of pain day after day with no break is the worst possible torture! I can't stop thinking that I'm his mother...I should be able to make his pain go away...I should be able to help my son - somehow. But there's no one who seems to know how to guide us! I feel like I can't breathe...like I can't move...like I can't function. Is anyone out there? We need help!

Desperate to find help for our son, Sander and I began looking for specialists around the country who treated CRPS. Our research elicited a few promising names, but even with my physical therapy training and Sander's medical background, it was confusing trying to make sense of the very different treatment approaches advocated by different doctors.

One theory suggested intense and aggressive physical therapy to push kids through the pain, past their point of tolerance, in order to basically override their nervous systems.

Another theory suggested a much more minimal approach with regular but mild physical therapy geared toward keeping the child functional and taking part in normal activities whenever possible. This theory implied that if you elicited too much pain, you could cause a "wind-up" phenomenon to occur whereby the central nervous system became sensitized and overexcited and the pain became embedded in the brain and thus harder to eliminate.

I already knew it was a fine line between pushing Devin to get through his exercises and triggering a horrible pain response that lasted for days. If I overdid it, he was incapacitated to the point of lying on the couch for the rest of the evening and missing school the next day, but if I lightened up on the exercises, he didn't make any progress or gain any strength.

After a great deal of research, Sander and I became intrigued by a pediatric pain specialist in Wisconsin who treated CRPS in children and teens. After discussing Devin's condition with him on the phone, we felt comfortable making the long trip to Wisconsin for a complete assessment by him and his team.

Leaving our home state in order to see a specialist was sobering, but I was excited that Devin was going to be evaluated by someone who specialized in this devastating and elusive neurological condition. With a diagnosis and proper treatment, we might actually see a light at the end of this tunnel.

*   *   *

One week before we were to leave, Devin inexplicably received a fresh injury at school. On his way from one class to another, as one of his buddies was giving him a piggyback ride to ensure he would make it to math on time, a student Devin didn't even know performed a powerful flying karate kick, hitting Devin's buttock at the exact site of his original injury. Devin fell hard to the ground, landing on his sore tailbone in excruciating pain. This random, impulsive act was pure bad luck; Devin simply happened to be in the wrong place at the wrong time on this particular day.

One urgent phone call later, I rushed to school and found Devin uncharacteristically in tears, refusing to put the slightest bit of weight on his leg. His pain had skyrocketed to a 10+ and the only way I could get him to the car was by wheelchair.

He was extremely uncomfortable and agitated, but I decided to leave the wheelchair at school and stop at a medical supply store on our way home for a pair of crutches. My plan was to have him slowly begin putting weight back on his right leg with assistance from the crutch. The longer he stayed off his leg, no matter how painful it was, the worse the situation would become.

After three long, difficult days, Devin was able to return to school with his still heightened level of pain and a new pair of crutches. Counting the days to our appointment in Wisconsin, I silently asked myself, "Can this nightmare get any worse?"

Little did I know how much I was tempting the fates.

*   *   *

On our way to Wisconsin, we stopped in Chicago to attend my nephew's bar mitzvah. The traveling was hard on Devin, and maneuvering through crowds of people on his crutches was equally tough. After he was bumped numerous times and experienced one minor fall, I gave in again and temporarily let him use a wheelchair.

I kept it to myself, but I was getting more and more worried. The longer Devin didn't use his leg, the more it would weaken, but he was still leery of putting weight on it. Thank heavens we were on our way to see a specialist. We needed help, and it couldn't come soon enough.

* * *

Upon our arrival at the children's hospital in Wisconsin, Devin and I located the main reception desk and then slowly made our way to the pain clinic on the 6th floor. Within moments of checking in, we were taken back to a lovely room with plush couches, lounge chairs and fresh flowers beautifully arranged on a table, where we spent a solid hour with the doctor, a nurse, and a social worker going over his history. This was gratifying, but for some reason I began to feel strangely ill at ease.

Have you ever felt that someone was hearing only what they wanted to hear in order to validate an already pre-determined judgment about you? That's how this experience felt, and I wasn't sure why. Maybe little smiles at the wrong time, or brief shakes of their heads, or even a few instances where, without me realizing it at the time, words were subtly put in my mouth.

After our initial meeting, Devin was taken away to be evaluated by the doctor and a physical therapist while I talked alone with the social worker. As I anxiously waited for them to return and give their diagnosis and recommendations, I decided I was just paranoid because of our recent bad experience with the specialist back home. This was an experienced and enthusiastic team with great knowledge about CRPS; surely we were in good hands.

When the doctor and therapist returned from evaluating Devin, I learned I wasn't paranoid at all. Solemnly, they told me Devin's pain was psychosomatic and that he was receiving some kind of secondary gain from pretending to be in pain. Perhaps he was looking for attention because of an emotional insecurity we were unaware of? In any event, he didn't have CRPS.

For a brief moment, I thought they must be joking. As I scanned their faces, I realized they were not, and immediately became thankful Devin wasn't in the room.

It wasn't easy, but I remained calm and reminded the doctor and therapist they were evaluating Devin after an acute re-injury to his nerve root at the original site of the injury. I reminded them that, since this recent incident a week ago, he'd been intensely fearful of putting any weight on that leg or letting anyone touch it. I told them that up until that point, Devin had been slow and in a lot of pain, but had walked everywhere with no assistive device.

The doctor responded that Devin had completely buckled when asked to stand on his right leg. He said this was a tell-tale sign he was faking his pain because even paraplegics can put weight on their legs by using their ligaments to support themselves.

He added that at the time of the examination, Devin's leg showed no color or temperature changes, whereas one of the telltale signs of CRPS is a red swollen limb with either hot or cold temperature changes.

I was flabbergasted. From my reading, I knew that color changes are indeed a telltale sign of CRPS, but also that these color and temperature changes come and go as part of the syndrome.

I explained that, more often than not, Devin's right leg was bright red and freezing. I also tried to explain that Devin was *afraid* to put weight on that leg, not incapable of doing it, but my explanations were in vain.

Momentarily, it flashed through my head that if what we'd endured with Devin over the last six months was all in his head, he had some very serious psychiatric problems.

Almost immediately, my instincts refuted this. The doctor and therapist were wrong, plain and simple, and anger surged within me. How dare they make this assumption about Devin? How dare they not take into consideration what had happened a week ago, how fearful he was of putting even the slightest bit of weight on his leg? How dare they ignore the well-known fact that color and temperature changes are often sporadic in patients with CRPS?

In spite of the emotions raging within me, I calmly told the doctor that I had a hard time believing Devin was faking his pain because he was a very happy and stable young man with many friends, interests, and a good family environment.

The doctor's reply was classic. He looked at me patiently and said, "I don't mean to be rude, but this is what all moms say to me."

He elaborated that this type of situation often occurs when kids feel too much pressure or experience family issues such as divorce or on-going marital problems.

I told him that Devin was an avid tennis player and crazy about the sport, that he would never do anything to interfere with what he loves. I explained that his father and I were very much in love and that Devin had an excellent relationship with his brother and sister, as well as a large group of friends who adored him.

The doctor just repeated, "I'm sorry, Wendy, but this is what all moms say to me."

I was obviously confused and upset, and finally he told me that Devin might have CRPS, but he couldn't make this diagnosis on the basis of Devin's current presentation.

In retrospect, I think he said this just to shut me up.

The doctor recommended changing Devin's pain medication to something called Lyrica in the hopes that Devin would have fewer side effects than with Neurontin. Almost as an aside, he commented that he'd never seen anyone have visual problems on Neurontin or Lyrica and that this symptom was all in Devin's head as well.

Once again, I was astounded. He thought Devin was faking visual blurriness? Plus, if he thought Devin was faking his pain, why was he giving him a prescription to control it? I was getting very mixed messages, and I felt sick to my stomach.

The doctor also recommended that Devin begin cognitive behavioral therapy. Not only would this help him deal with his pain, he explained, it would uncover the secondary gain he was receiving from subconsciously pretending to be in pain.

Finally, the doctor wanted Devin to continue his strict physical therapy program, but without any input from me. Under the circumstances, he told me, my being an experienced physical therapist was more a hindrance than a help.

I had no problem with another physical therapist taking charge of Devin's exercise program – it would be difficult for any parent to stay objective while her child endured severe pain – but to come to the conclusion that I was an impediment to Devin's recovery was completely out of line. Most doctors, when they learned I was a physical therapist, said how lucky Devin was to have a parent who understood the dynamics of exercise and could monitor an exercise program at home.

Quickly, I realized I had two choices: I could tell the doctor this was the most ridiculous thing I'd ever heard and he didn't know what he was talking about, or I could try not to overreact, be as mature as possible, and actually try to listen to what he was saying. Devin's situation was worsening, we'd traveled a long way to see this physician, and CRPS was his specialty. I wouldn't be doing Devin any favors if I let my pride get in the way of curing him, and if there was even a grain of truth to what he said, I needed to know it.

In hindsight, it is clear I made the wrong choice. I should have remembered: *mothers always know best.* Deep in my heart, I knew this doctor was wrong. I should have trusted my instincts, but this is hard to do when times are desperate. Sander and I had been floundering with failed treatments for months, increasingly desperate to find the answer to Devin's deteriorating condition. As maddening as it was to hear that this team of professionals believed Devin's pain was psychosomatic, at that moment, I felt I had no choice but to entertain the implausible concept that maybe it *was* all in our son's head.

*   *   *

Against my better judgment, I made an agreement with the doctor. He would be Devin's sole physician, and Sander and I would ignore anything and everything related to Devin's pain. We would act as if everything were all right and not ask Devin how he was doing, ever. In addition, we would do nothing to help him with his mobility, even if he were in pain.

To be honest, this part of the agreement wasn't a problem. We did no more for Devin than we did for our other two children because we knew it was important to keep him walking and functional. Likewise, we rarely asked Devin about his pain. All parents know that dwelling on it, particularly with kids, can make the situation worse.

It wasn't so easy agreeing with the doctor's final caveat: that under no circumstances, no matter how much pain he was in, was Devin to leave school.

Just thinking about this made tears come to my eyes. Try explaining this concept to the teachers or principal when they knew Devin was suffering and needed to spend the day at home. The only way to comprehend this was if you believed Devin was faking his pain, and we knew otherwise.

As reluctant as I was, I followed this doctor's advice. Confused, sick at heart, and increasingly depressed, I left the appointment questioning myself and everything I knew about my son.

*   *   *

The Wisconsin doctor didn't share with Devin his view that Devin's pain was psychosomatic. Instead, he chose to tell him that although his pain was real, his mind was playing tricks on him. He told Devin he had a form of CRPS and emphasized that physical therapy and continuing his daily activities, including not leaving school, were crucial. He also told Devin he wanted him to see a therapist for counseling.

Devin was uncharacteristically silent at this meeting. He asked no questions of the doctor, and he looked puzzled and uncomfortable.

Trying to recap what we'd heard once we were back in the car was challenging. I tried my best to hide that I was upset, but Devin knew something wasn't right.

"Do I really have CRPS?" he asked. "Why does he think my brain is playing tricks on me, and why does he want me to see a therapist?"

I had no intention of sharing the doctor's real opinion about

Devin's condition. What a slap in the face it would have been, after six months of suffering, to be told, "He doesn't believe in you" and "Your pain isn't real."

What's more, as his parent, it was important that Devin know *I* believed him, and if I did, why was I following this doctor's advice? Devin's trust in his father and me and his belief that we would find a way to make his pain go away was too important to sacrifice.

Somehow, I pulled a rabbit out of my hat. I told Devin the doctor thought he had CRPS, but since his leg wasn't red and cold today, he couldn't be 100% certain. Nonetheless, he was still going to treat Devin as if he had CRPS, with physical therapy and medicine, since this was his best guess.

"As far as your mind playing tricks on you," I told him, "this was the doctor's way of explaining how your nervous system is sending pain messages to your brain even though your original injury to the nerve root has healed."

In essence, this was exactly what was happening, although this wasn't how the doctor had meant it.

"The counseling," I explained, "is to help you deal with the daily struggles of suffering from this type of pain."

This explanation seemed to placate Devin, but he was obviously still uneasy. On an intuitive level, he knew something wasn't right.

Meanwhile, I couldn't keep my mind from wandering. *Could* my son have a psychological disorder that caused him to believe he was in severe pain?

As quickly as that thought would surface, I would bury it deep and replace it with anger at myself for entertaining such an idea, as well as fury at the physician for not believing Devin and for making such generalizations about our family.

In spite of my swirling thoughts, I managed to talk to my son with a smile on my face as I confidently relayed to him that the exercises and the new medicine would make a difference.

Clearly, I was an emotional wreck.

*   *   *

Once we returned home, Devin began to see a respected cognitive behavioral therapist in our home community. Our son wasn't shy about telling us he thought it was a big waste of time, but he agreed to give it a try.

After eight straight weeks of treating Devin, the therapist's conclusion was balm to our souls. He told us Devin was an extremely mature, stable kid with an excellent support system who was handling his pain better than most adults would. He saw no secondary gain whatsoever and said it was unnecessary to continue seeing Devin; he would only need to be seen if he wanted to talk with someone about his pain.

As thrilled as I was to hear this, I begged the therapist to see Devin a few more times to be certain he couldn't find any underlying secondary gain.

The therapist agreed, but four visits later, he repeated the same conclusion: there was no core psychological justification for the pain. In his opinion, Devin wasn't faking it.

At that, we discontinued his services, glad we had pursued this therapy because it might have helped, fully confident that it was appropriate to put our time and energy into other forms of treatment.

*   *   *

During this exhausting and demoralizing eight-week period, it became obvious to us that Devin's condition was continuing to deteriorate and that the new medication, Lyrica, was inadequate to control his pain. Many days, he spent hours lying on the cot in the nursing office at school after being injured or when he couldn't tolerate sitting in class. I often received urgent phone calls from a distraught secretary telling me how uncomfortable Devin was and pleading with me to let him come home.

With tears in my eyes, I had to say I was sorry, but his doctor wanted him to stay at school. Each call tore me apart inside, and I have to say, I'm sure the school personnel were beginning to question my judgment.

Finally, Devin begged his father and me to ask the Wisconsin doctor to either change his medication or increase the dose. His pain was becoming unbearable, and he was pleading for our help.

During our phone call, the specialist agreed to up Devin's Lyrica. He told me 600 mg was a high dose for a child Devin's age, but assured me Devin could handle it.

The higher dose did help a bit more, but it also caused Devin to become tremendously lightheaded and nauseous. Shortly after he started the new dosage, he actually fainted a couple of times in the bathroom at the junior high, only to be found by a teacher or another student passed out in a stall. In one of these instances, I was frantically called by the school secretary and told that Devin had a seizure and to come immediately! After sorting things out with the nurse, we discovered that Devin had felt sick to his stomach and was extremely dizzy while walking to the bathroom where he fainted while kneeling next to the toilet. It was obvious that Devin was going to require an escort throughout the day during school, and we set this in place immediately.

The increased dose worsened his vision, too, as well as his ability to process information. On top of this, after about 10 days on the higher dose, he began to vomit. At first we thought he had the flu, but after five days of not being able to keep even the tiniest morsel of food down, I began to wonder if he was reacting to the medication.

I got back on the web, and not only did I discover that 600 mg of Lyrica is truly a large dose for a boy Devin's size, I also read, way at the bottom of the list, about possible side effects including nausea and vomiting.

I called the doctor, and his response was in keeping with his attitude, approach, and care of Devin all along.

"Wendy, this is all part of Devin's psychosomatic response. It's the same as his pain. It basically doesn't exist, and he's getting some secondary gain from this behavior."

My ears literally rang. Was I hearing him correctly? Devin was vomiting, had lost 10 pounds, and hadn't eaten for almost a week for *attention?* Like he hadn't gotten enough attention already?

The doctor responded adamantly that this problem, like the blurry vision Devin was reporting, was not a side effect of the Lyrica.

I replied that I'd read up on the medicine and that both blurry vision and nausea could be side effects.

His response was classic: "I have never seen this happen, so it isn't true."

I hung up and called a local gastroenterologist. As a favor to my husband, he agreed to see Devin that same day. Without delay, we hopped in the car and drove to his busy office where he kindly squeezed Devin in between patients. After examining him and hearing the story, he swiftly concluded that Devin's severe queasiness was a result of the high dose of Lyrica.

I told him this was exactly my gut feeling, but that his current doctor said this couldn't be the case because he'd never seen it happen.

Later that afternoon, just to be certain there were no lesions that might be responsible for the vomiting, the gastroenterologist had us return to his surgical clinic where he scoped Devin. Under anesthesia, a tube with a camera attached to its end was placed down Devin's throat and funneled through his esophagus to his stomach.

After the procedure, the doctor met with us, confirmed the scope was clean, and once again recommended weaning Devin from the Lyrica. I thanked him for seeing Devin on such short notice and for his sound advice, then took my emaciated and exhausted son back home.

Sure enough, over the next few days, as we lowered the dose back to 450 mg, Devin's nausea subsided and he began to eat.

It was then that it hit me: Devin's so-called specialist didn't know what he was doing. He didn't know our son. He'd made a gross generalization based on a cursory evaluation and was leading us in the wrong direction. Since entering his care, Devin's already poor condition had deteriorated, and so had my frame of mind. I'd spent these past weeks in an angry state of disbelief, feeling lost, depressed, and irritated with myself for following a treatment approach that deep inside I knew was terribly wrong. Worst of all, we'd wasted two precious months because I'd ignored rather than trusted my instincts.

Suddenly, the despair and depression I'd felt since our trip to Wisconsin began to dissipate. Devin was hurting and needed help. I knew in my heart he had CRPS, no matter what this so-called specialist said. There were other doctors who could help us, and I wasn't going to waste any more time.

* * *

Sander began to steal an hour of time here and there at the office and I used every free minute I could find to once again scour the internet. We even put our sleepless nights to good use, googling everything and anything that could possibly be helpful to Devin. We already knew the basics about CRPS from our prior research, but now we devoured everything we could find.

Over and over, we read how important the six-month to one-year mark was. Virtually every article stated that the sooner you can find a treatment that works, the more likely it is you can cure this disease.

Unfortunately, we also found literature claiming CRPS becomes harder to control after the first year, as well as a number of papers that discuss how frequently patients see doctors who don't believe their pain is real. The advice of these authors was to keep searching until you find the right physician.

Such validation and encouragement was very gratifying. I only wish I'd trusted my instincts back in Wisconsin. I wish I'd chosen to walk away right then and there and look for another opinion. To this day, I feel guilty for having even a speck of doubt about my son, and I am still angry when I think about this period of time and about this doctor.

I wanted desperately to confront him about his faulty assessment and inappropriate recommendations for our son, but Sander dissuaded me, and in hindsight I am grateful. It was best to take a deep breath, put it behind me, and move on, so that is exactly what I did.

We were at six months now since Devin's original injury, and the clock was ticking. I set aside my anger as well as my private feelings of guilt and once again channeled my energy into finding an answer.

Chapter 4

Back on Track and Looking for Answers

April 19, 2008

5:30 a.m. Another sleepless night. I'm getting used to these. At least I'm productive, though tonight it took me a good 45 minutes of crying like a baby to realize I wasn't doing Devin any good in this pathetic state. After I uncurled myself from my tightly wound fetal position, blew my nose, and got a bowl of Apple Jacks, I spent almost three hours on the internet researching everything I could find on CRPS.

Man, every time I get online I find new bits of information. The problem is, it's so hard to decipher what's useful and put it all together in a meaningful way. Why can't I find a basic protocol anywhere? All I seem to be finding are tons of conflicting opinions on the same treatments. Nothing is coordinated! Yuck! This is going to be much harder than I ever imagined. Unfortunately, Sander and I have no choice except to figure it out...quickly!

I'm keeping good notes tonight...Gonna try to catch a few winks before the kids wake up.

One of my first decisions after discontinuing our services with the Wisconsin doctor was to up the ante on Devin's therapy and exercise routine. Though he was seeing a different physical therapist two to three times a week and followed my home exercise program another three days each week, he wasn't getting anywhere because of our ambivalence about how hard to push.

With my concern over his weakening leg paramount and the distance to his physical therapy appointments becoming more and more burdensome, I decided I would provide a more intense program right from home. Tiptoeing around his pain wasn't working, so I would push much harder, building strength and endurance very slowly, yet requiring new goals to be reached on a weekly basis.

Devin's new plan consisted of exercising multiple times throughout the day as well as working as hard as he could right through the pain. Specifically, he swam each morning at 6:00 a.m. before school, did strength training and stretching each day after school, and rode the stationary bike every evening for 15 minutes.

Each day, a kitchen timer in hand, I counted the seconds he could tolerate standing on his right leg. I used a ruler to measure the distance he could raise his right leg or hip off the floor while in different positions lying on the ground. I required him to increase the amount of his leg weights by one half pound each week as well as the number of repetitions he performed with each exercise. I asked him to increase his time or resistance as he rode the stationary bike each evening and the number of laps he swam each morning.

It was painful, but the buoyancy and non-weight-bearing component of the water allowed him to tolerate swimming laps fairly well. My job was to coach him from the side of the pool and remind him to kick and use his right leg with each stroke he took.

I stayed positive and encouraging to Devin, but I struggled every day with my role. Driven by some combination of my physical therapy training and pure instinct, I was basically using the concept of desensitization that we would later embrace with every fiber of our beings. I was still fearful about triggering a terrible flare, but I also felt that if he could work through it, maybe his body would start accepting the sensation as tolerable.

To his credit, Devin was fully committed to this new, more intense exercise program, even though it took about two hours each day to complete. He desperately wanted his pain gone and his life back, so he was willing to endure whatever I threw at him.

Nonetheless, completing his daily program was slow, tedious, and extremely painful. Just the simple act of bearing weight on his right leg without the support of his left leg for more than three seconds caused tears to stream down his face. These sessions didn't fully incapacitate him, but he was always a bit worse for wear afterwards, and so was I.

All the while, I was working with the principal at Devin's junior high to arrange a 504 plan for him. Section 504 of the Rehabilitation Act and the Americans with Disabilities Act requires schools to offer accommodations and modifications to students with certain disabilities to keep them functional and help them be successful at school.

In Devin's case, the 504 plan gave him the flexibility to be able to spend additional time in therapy by eliminating all unnecessary classes and electives. It allowed him to arrive at school one hour late each morning, after he swam, and leave one hour early each afternoon, which allowed him to complete his strengthening and stretching program before his brother and sister got out of school.

Without the 504 plan, a large portion of Devin's program would have been squeezed into the late afternoon and evening and I would never have been able to keep up with my household obligations or Ethan and Taylor's extracurricular activities. It was tight, but if we stayed structured, I could provide my other two children with well deserved attention and we could preserve some semblance of normalcy in our lives.

Once he was fully independent and didn't require my coaching from the side of the pool, Taylor and I made the best of our early morning situation by checking out each and every breakfast establishment in our little town while Devin swam and showered. It was nice to have this one-on-one time together before I dropped her off at school. Taylor, very mature for her age, seemed to be doing fine, but the stress of watching her brother suffer for so long was taking its toll.

In spite of our best efforts, Devin's pain regularly consumed our household like a thick fog. So many times, we would be sitting at dinner or playing a game together around the coffee table when someone would accidentally bump Devin's right leg or Maggie, our large Portuguese water dog, would lightly paw him.

Devin would let out a terrific scream and, with a tear streaking down his cheek, retreat into his quiet world of agony. There wasn't anything we could do to help him. As a family, we lived on a bed of eggshells. Day in and day out, we silently worried about Devin's suffering and waited for the ground to crack open beneath him each time he was hurt.

The only positive at this time was that I was actively helping my son once again. I actively believed in my son once again. The core rightness of this gave me the strength to keep going.

* * *

As Sander and I continued our pursuit of specialists and potential treatments, we began to wonder if an in-patient pediatric rehabilitation pain program might be the answer. Providing treatment as an in-patient sounded radical, but maybe this was the only way to control Devin's pain.

Each program involved admitting him to the hospital for interventions such as spinal blocks, which he'd already unsuccessfully tried, and intrathecal catheters, thin tubes surgically placed next to the spinal cord through which analgesic medicines are administered. These programs also offered medication trials and support groups, and the doctors would help prepare a care plan before Devin was discharged.

We made appointments for Devin to receive an initial evaluation with doctors from two different programs, the Cleveland Clinic and the Children's Hospital at Johns Hopkins.

To our dismay, the earliest appointments we could get were at the beginning of the summer, and the waiting lists to get into the programs themselves were even longer. Optimistically, we hoped for a miracle that would catapult Devin to the top of these extremely long lists. Our goal was to have his pain under control by the end of the summer so that when school began in the fall, he could begin his freshman year of high school in good shape.

At this point, in spite of our collective best efforts and his 504 plan, he was barely passing the eighth grade. More importantly, his pain, his missed days at school, and the continued side effects of his pain medication meant he hadn't learned much this year. We needed to resolve all this before he entered high school.

As spring passed and we anxiously waited for our appointments in Cleveland and Baltimore, my husband received an unexpected phone call from our sister-in-law, a gynecologist in California. A patient of hers with CRPS was seeing a neurologist from the San Francisco area named Dr. Chagnon. This patient claimed Dr. Chagnon had great knowledge about CRPS and had helped control her pain. Our sister-in-law suggested we contact Dr. Chagnon just to see what she had to say.

As an aside, she wondered if we'd considered acupuncture for Devin. She was a great believer in this ancient Chinese art of healing and basically asked, "What could it hurt?"

*   *   *

A little research sparked my curiosity, and as Sander attempted to make contact with Dr. Chagnon, I decided to contact a well-known acupuncturist in our area. I'd always been a skeptic of acupuncture, but now I hoped I would be miserably put to shame.

Accordingly, we walked into the acupuncturist's office the following week with open minds. Impressively, she had researched CRPS prior to our visit and had even consulted her mentors about the best way to treat Devin.

I was taken aback by her enthusiasm and honest interest in helping him. She was optimistic we would see results, and she described the concept of energy fields that exist throughout our bodies before presenting us with a diagram of a curled-up fetus situated snuggly within a picture of an ear.

"This," she explained, "is an energy map of the body."

My skepticism slowly returned. I couldn't help but tell her this made no medical sense to me.

With a kind smile, she said, "Some things are never meant to be fully understood," and led Devin and me back into a small room.

She directed me to a chair in the corner and had Devin lie face up on the table. She placed small needles in certain areas of his ears and hands that correlated to the energy map she had shown us, dimmed the lights, told Devin to relax, and said she'd be back in 20 minutes or so.

After a couple of minutes in the dark, Devin said, "Mom, are my legs supposed to be getting warm?"

Intrigued, I told him to just relax and to see what happened over the next 15 minutes.

Upon her return, the acupuncturist was thrilled to hear that Devin's leg had experienced a warm sensation, even though his pain hadn't changed. She added a few more needles to his hands and we waited another 15 minutes, but Devin reported the same results.

The acupuncturist told us not to be discouraged. She was happy he'd had any response, and said it could take five or six more visits before he felt any relief.

Devin and I thanked her and left her office with a new respect for the field of acupuncture. How cool that those little needles in his ear could cause a warming sensation to his legs! For the life of me, I couldn't figure out how, but that was okay. We were both excited to see what the next five visits would bring.

Unfortunately, after seven total visits, Devin's pain never budged. Disappointed but not upset with our decision to try, we checked acupuncture off our list. It didn't work for Devin, but it certainly opened my mind to the benefits this treatment could have on other medical conditions.

*   *   *

Sander took his sister's advice. In May, eight months after Devin's original injury, he called Dr. Chagnon and left her a message. She thoughtfully returned Sander's call that same day, and they chatted for over 45 minutes.

Sander was impressed with her willingness to discuss Devin's situation at length as well as her vast knowledge about CRPS. She seemed to have endless ideas, and she conveyed to Sander her belief that, assuming Devin had CRPS, we should be looking for a cure for him rather than accepting that he had a chronic condition that required palliative care. Most literature we'd read indicates there's no cure for CRPS, but Dr. Chagnon told Sander her personal experience suggested otherwise. She felt we were early enough to shoot for a cure, and she noted that children and teens often had a full recovery if the problem was caught soon enough.

She was appalled to hear about our experience with the doctor in Wisconsin and said it's common to find doctors who don't believe pain is real. Although she wasn't familiar with the two pediatric pain programs we had appointments with, she was a bit leery of some of the in-patient pediatric pain programs and suggested we be careful when choosing one. She explained that some are less individualized than others and many are palliative. She emphasized again that we should avoid helping Devin *deal* with the pain and instead concentrate on curing him completely.

After receiving Devin's complete history, she e-mailed us back with a slew of suggestions including the placement of an intrathecal catheter as an in-patient with the goal of providing temporary but complete pain relief in order to re-set the brain. She also described the benefits of numerous other treatment options, including intravenous bisphosphonate, a cutting-edge drug that works to reuptake excess calcium (one of the culprits in CRPS), and intravenous solumedral drip, a powerful anti-inflammatory agent.

She also suggested the possibility of using oral ketamine, a strong hallucinogen that acts to block the N-methyl D-aspartate (NMDA) receptors of the spinal cord and brain. Simplistically, the NMDA receptors are the main neural receptors in the pain pathway that bind glutamate. They are responsible for opening the gate and allowing the pain signal to travel through the spinal cord to the brain.

Her email also described numerous medication trials Devin could participate in, including using snail toxins as a form of analgesia, along with a careful description of each medication and the physiologic rational for its use. The list was so extensive, it was mind-boggling, and we immediately felt a sense of hope.

Dr. Chagnon strongly believed in trying to prevent the "wind-up" phenomenon from occurring. She felt that the more pain a patient endured over a long period of time, the more likely the brain could interpret this as a normal sensation that became permanently imprinted within the central nervous system.

Her vehement opinion on this topic worried me, given the intense therapy Devin was currently involved in and the acute pain it caused, and I set up an hour-long phone evaluation so that I, too, could hear her ideas.

Like Sander, I was amazed at Dr. Chagnon's immense knowledge about this condition. She further explained to me the theoretical biomedical basis for CRPS, the actual receptor involved, the neurological pathway, and the chemical and cellular involvement. She had thoroughly researched this disease and had a huge knowledge base from which to work, with a seemingly endless "bag of tricks" as treatment options. Most importantly, she listened carefully to Devin's story, believed he had CRPS, and felt there was a cure in his future.

After our discussion, I asked if we could bring Devin to her hospital in Sonoma and admit him as an in-patient under her care over the summer to try some of her treatment suggestions. I told her she was exactly the type of physician we'd been looking for. She had the knowledge, the experience, the compassion, and most importantly the belief in Devin and the confidence in a cure. Why would we go anywhere else?

Dr. Chagnon had just relocated to Sonoma from a large hospital in San Francisco where the set-up for this type of care was already in place. She said the hospital in Sonoma was extremely small, but if we could be patient, she would pull together a team of anesthesiologists, nurses, and physical therapists to make it happen.

As a result, we cancelled our appointments with the other two pain programs. While we waited impatiently for the phone call from Dr. Chagnon telling us we could make the trip to California, we continued Devin's new physical therapy program. In spite of Dr. Chagnon's concerns regarding the wind-up phenomenon, I couldn't bear to see him stagnate over the next several months.

*   *   *

Summer came, and we deliberately put the pressures of school and Devin's cognitive and visual issues behind us for a much-needed reprieve.

Each day, Devin worked hard with his exercises. Soon, he began to accomplish small and very specific goals. He could now stand on his right leg for six seconds. He could ride the stationary bike for 15 minutes at 1.7 mph. He could lift his right leg 13 inches off the ground while lying flat on his back. It wasn't much, but we were actually starting to make a little progress.

It happened to be a beautiful summer in northern Michigan. In addition to Devin's exercises, our days were filled with afternoons at the beach, hiking with Taylor and her friends up the Sleeping Bear Sand Dunes, sailing and kayaking, late-night bonfires, and visits from out-of-town family and friends. Summers in northern Michigan are always rejuvenating, but knowing we were about to see the doctor who believed she could help Devin become pain free made this particular couple of months especially therapeutic.

In addition to our routine summer bliss, Taylor enjoyed two weeks of fun at an overnight camp, which happened to be the same camp where Ethan was working as a counselor, and they both had a ball.

In mid-July, we even allowed Devin to join his father on their annual fly-fishing excursion to Yellowstone National Park. Like his dad, Devin could spend day after day, hour after hour, fishing the majestic rivers of this national park, oblivious to bear and bison lurking on all sides. In mutual bliss, they invariably lost track of time and had to pull one another off the river.

We were hesitant about sending Devin this particular summer, but the lure of fly fishing and fond memories of spending this special time with his father convinced him he should try.

In retrospect, we should have known better. After his first few hours wading within the brisk rivers, Devin was begging his father to take him back to their rustic cabin. He spent most of the rest of the trip lying uncomfortably in bed in Silvertree, Montana, with no television, listening to his iPod hour after hour.

Upon their return to Traverse City, he spent the rest of the summer hanging out with friends, relaxing, playing the piano, and waiting to go to California.

We also resumed his exercise program, and by early August, though he still sported an impressive limp, he was walking just a little bit better.

This was encouraging, but his pain hadn't budged. His attitude remained good, but prior to our trip to Sonoma, his pain still hovered at a 7 to 7 ½ and he was still incapacitated if anyone touched his leg, however lightly.

I have to admit, as our California plans solidified, I began to get nervous about how hard I'd been pushing him. Guiltily, I eased off a bit, especially on the exercises that were the most painful. Dr. Chagnon was cautious about facilitating too much pain, and I wanted to respect this as Devin entered her care.

Chapter 5

Our Trip to the Wine Country

August 6, 2008

Devin is sound asleep. Not surprising after our long day. We had two transfers from Traverse City to San Francisco through Chicago and Dallas. I wasn't looking forward to one airport, much less two big ones, especially since Devin didn't want to use a wheelchair. He insisted on walking the entire length of these huge terminals all day long. Luckily, we had very long layovers, so I told him to go for it if he could. His pace – at the speed of a severely injured turtle – was highlighted by the people whizzing by us on their way to their connections. It was a ridiculous sight, and he had to stop every 50 feet or so for a break because of his pain. One lady, not so nicely, asked me why I was making him walk in his condition. Anyway, we're here! Can't wait to meet Dr. Chagnon tomorrow!

Sonoma sits smack dab in the middle of California's wine country amidst beautiful rolling hills and vineyards. Equal parts excited and apprehensive, Devin and I flew into San Francisco on August 6 and rented a car. Our leisurely drive, as the sun was beginning to set over the countryside, was extraordinarily beautiful. "This is a good omen," I told myself.

We arrived in the quaint town of Sonoma just as evening was settling in. It was easy to locate the hospital even in the dark, and we effortlessly found a hotel just around the corner and settled in for the night.

The first item on our agenda the next morning was to locate a piano at a church or community hall that Devin could play while he was here. This too required little effort, and we quickly had the choice of two different churches that kindly opened their doors to Devin anytime he wanted.

In his element, Devin entertained the clergy and random congregants throughout the day, improvising to his favorite jazz pieces like "My Funny Valentine" and "Sentimental Mood" and inspiring them with "Rachmaninoff Piano Concerto No. 2 in C Minor" until it was time to meet Dr. Chagnon.

My relief was palpable when we finally met this doctor who had taken such a great interest in Devin and seemed to know so much about his condition. Although her office was very busy that day, she spent a long time welcoming us to Sonoma, making sure we had good accommodations, getting to know Devin, and performing a full evaluation. With confidence, she confirmed the diagnosis of CRPS.

Her first suggestion was to try a bilateral sympathetic block. Devin's other sympathetic blocks had been performed on only one side of his spinal column, and she explained how crossover of nerve transmission occurs within the spinal cord, which might explain why this procedure hadn't been effective.

Devin received this procedure the same day as an out-patient in the operating room at Sonoma Valley Hospital. It resulted in little pain relief, so Dr. Chagnon decided to immediately admit him to the ICU for an intrathecal catheter to be placed in his spine. This type of catheter administers strong medications and opiates to the nerves in the spinal column and requires close monitoring, but would block the pain in Devin's right leg.

Once he was completely pain free, Dr. Chagnon felt intensive physical therapy could begin without the worry of triggering a flare-up. Her secondary goal was to maintain this zero pain level for a period of five to seven days in the hopes of resetting Devin's nervous system.

Now that I knew the game plan, I found an apartment to rent

above the garage of a lovely family a half mile from the hospital. We expected Devin to be an inpatient for approximately one week and then to remain as an outpatient for another week or so. At the end of this period, hopefully pain free, he would return home and continue the intense physical therapy that would bring his leg back to its former strength.

Two weeks was a long time to be gone, but given the lengthy and fruitless efforts we'd already expended, it seemed like a small price to pay. Sander, Ethan, and Taylor were enjoying the waning days of summer swimming and boating in beautiful East Grand Traverse Bay right across the street from our home, and I had additional peace of mind knowing Sander's entire family would be visiting while we were gone.

His parents and sister's family from Detroit and his brother's family, ironically from northern California, had joined us every year since the kids were babies. Numerous photo albums show us tubing down the Crystal River, hiking to Pyramid Point, picnicking on the bluffs of Lake Michigan, playing mini golf, racing down water slides, and enjoying priceless family time at nightly bonfires on the beach.

It was a shame we had to miss the fun, but Sander would have a week off from work and Taylor would be fully attended to by loving cousins, aunts, uncles, and of course her grandparents.

Before our departure, I'd made certain all three kids were ready for school. I'd purchased the necessary clothes and supplies, and I'd even provided Sander with detailed instructions describing the many other nuances of our busy household and the kids' daily routines. Taylor's soccer practice schedule was posted on the refrigerator and various carpools were prearranged. I certainly hoped we'd be back before school started, but if there was one thing Devin's elusive illness had taught me, it was to prepare for anything.

* * *

Dr. Chagnon had arranged for an experienced anesthesiologist to surgically place Devin's intrathecal catheter. Unfortunately, even after it was inserted, Devin still felt quite a bit of pain. What's more, the medicine didn't reach all areas of his leg, so he was taken into surgery a second time the next day to replace it, with only a slightly better outcome.

The anesthesiologist, though experienced, hadn't worked much with CRPS. He was shocked that Devin still felt pain and noted that he was giving Devin a larger dose than he gave women in childbirth.

In response, Dr. Chagnon explained that a portion of Devin's pain was being mediated by the central nervous system and was therefore difficult to control.

All told, Devin went back to the operating room five times in seven days to try to place the catheter correctly to get full coverage of his right leg. Finally, on day seven, after placing a second catheter along with the first, Devin felt full coverage of the right leg. In practical terms, this meant he was completely paralyzed in his right leg and needed a walker to get to and from the bathroom.

Incredibly, despite the two catheters, loads of opiates, and the full coverage, he still felt a small sensation of pain in the leg, but Dr. Chagnon was happy to have gotten this far. She wanted to begin physical therapy immediately while his brain had a chance to reset.

During the next week as an inpatient at the hospital, Devin also received a strong steroid infusion for five days for the purpose of decreasing any residual inflammation in his spine and a bisphosphonate IV drip for three days. Dr. Chagnon had presented some very promising research indicating this calcium re-uptake agent helped eliminate excess calcium from the synaptic cleft within the spinal cord, which then slowed down further chemical reactions responsible for the transmission of pain signals to the brain.

As expected, these aggressive procedures were tough for Devin to endure. In addition to the discomfort from the five operating room visits and the placement of the spinal catheter, the medicines traveling through the catheter made him nauseous day and night. Making matters worse, as expected, the bisphosphonate drip caused a fever, full body aches, and severe shaking for three entire days.

For the icing on the cake, Dr. Chagnon was also giving Devin a daily liquid supplement used for pain relief that tasted like rotten eggs and continuing the trial of oral ketamine he'd begun taking two weeks prior to our arrival in Sonoma.

This powerful, controversial hallucinogen made me particularly nervous, but we hoped it would block the NMDA receptors in Devin's spinal cord responsible for allowing the transmission of pain signals to his brain.

"Special K," as it is known in some circles, is one of the infamous "date rape drugs" that has earned such a heinous reputation outside the operating room. Approved as an anesthetic for children in 1970 and used by veterinarians as a tranquilizer for horses, this drug has been compared to LSD and PCP and is serious stuff.

Long discussions with Dr. Chagnon about possible consequences and plenty of research of my own had revealed no known long-term effects of using ketamine for the treatment of pain, so Sander and I had reluctantly agreed to proceed.

The side effects weren't good – at home, this drug made Devin feel slightly high and very fatigued – but they were tolerable. Under Dr. Chagnon's care in the ICU, he began taking a higher dose of ketamine and his symptoms escalated.

One evening, he began having severe hallucinations. He felt like he couldn't breathe, his coordination became extremely impaired, his speech became slurred, and he began to have partial facial paralysis, which made drinking water very difficult. Worst of all, he became extremely anxious and kept saying, "Please make it stop; I don't like this!"

These disturbing effects peaked and then mostly disappeared within a few hours, but I was very shaken by what I'd seen. I felt like I had a front row seat from which to watch my son overdose on one of the world's most abominable drugs. Whether it helped or not, were the side effects worth it?

Later that night, when Devin was sound asleep, thanks to the heavy-duty sleeping medication he was taking, I went back to the apartment, sat in the dark and cried. All I could think was, "What the hell are we doing?"

Although the nurses and Dr. Chagnon were unbelievably understanding, caring, and accommodating, I began to second-guess our decision to attempt these invasive and extremely aggressive procedures.

"What if none of these procedures or medications work?" I asked Sander on the phone that night. "Is it worth the trauma we're putting Devin through?"

The next day, I told Dr. Chagnon we had to nix the oral ketamine. Even if it helped block his pain, I couldn't bear to watch Devin endure the side effects. Besides, in spite of the research I'd done, I couldn't help but fear that something this powerful could do long-term damage to his brain.

Dr. Chagnon understood my reservation, and without judgment she respected my decision to have Devin stop the oral ketamine.

*   *   *

Throughout this trying time, I kept to a strict schedule, which helped me keep my emotions and panic under control and present a brave face to Devin.

Each day, I awakened at 6:00 a.m., took a quick run through the vineyards, showered, then spent from 7:30 a.m. to 9:00 p.m. in the ICU with him. When he was able, we played cards and board games, saw way too many replays of beach volleyball tournaments on television from the Summer Olympics, and watched full seasons of *Heroes* and *Weeds*.

These activities and twice-daily food runs for him at lunch and dinner were the highlights of what turned out to be a 15-day stay in the ICU at Sonoma Valley Hospital. Although the plan was only to keep him in ICU for a week, the unanticipated delays caused by numerous return visits to the operating room in order to readjust the catheter extended his stay.

As the days dragged by, I truly felt lost and more than a bit pessimistic, but Devin's spirits stayed relatively good. In spite of the misery caused by the medications and the discomfort from the catheters, the pain in his right leg was almost nonexistent for the first time in a year, he was making friends with all his nurses, he had good music to listen to and entertaining DVD's to watch, and his every need was catered to by yours truly. A couple of times, when he felt up to it, he was even assisted to the geriatric floor, IVs in tow, where he was allowed to play the hospital's resident piano.

It was rather comical to hear him improvise to "Georgia on My Mind" and "Afternoon in Paris" in his skimpy hospital gown, un-groomed, un-showered, and hooked up to three IVs. Nonetheless, the nursing staff and a few patients commented that if they shut their eyes, they felt they were in a classy nightclub.

Overall, I felt very safe and comfortable under Dr. Chagnon's care; I just wasn't sure these aggressive procedures were going to work, and I couldn't help but wonder if they were worth the high price Devin was paying.

*   *   *

As expected, on day 15, when we slowly weaned Devin from the intrathecal catheter cocktail, his pain began to return. However, instead of the 7 -7 1/2 out of 10 he'd had when admitted, his pain was at a 6-6 1/2. This was nowhere as low as we wanted, but it was the first sign of progress we'd seen.

"CRPS is tough to break and often resistant to even the most aggressive treatment approaches," Dr. Chagnon reminded us. Devin had responded, and the bisphosphonate wouldn't fully kick in for almost a month, so more progress could hopefully be expected.

On August 21, the morning he was discharged, Dr. Chagnon scheduled an exotic animal trainer to visit the hospital with over a dozen exotic animals. I was very touched that she went to all this trouble for Devin. She really cared about him and desperately wanted to help him. He had experienced numerous hellish moments under her care, and she often told me how impressed she was with how he handled himself as he experienced the many uncomfortable side effects that came with the multitude of treatments he'd received.

Devin appreciated her efforts, but he was frantic to get back to the apartment for his first real shower in two weeks.

I say "real shower" because on the ninth day in the ICU, after begging the nurses, he had attempted to take a shower on the unit while sitting in his wheelchair. After only a few short minutes, the excess movement of his body and the difficulty keeping the surgical site dry had caused his catheter to slip out of place. Once again, he'd been whisked to surgery to replace the catheter. Not wishing for a repeat of this experience, I'd learned how to wash his hair while he lay in bed, and Devin had learned how to carefully sponge bathe behind a curtain.

We intended to return to the hospital to see the animals after he was cleaned up, but once he'd showered, he began to feel overwhelmingly fatigued. His back hurt from all the probing and surgical procedures, and he was so weak from not moving his leg for two-plus weeks that he could barely walk.

While he stayed at the apartment and slept for almost twelve hours, I returned to the hospital to see the animals, which were thoroughly enjoyed by the residents of the nursing floor. Everyone I met had heard about Devin and showered me with well wishes for him. This was a nice perk that came with being cared for in a small-town hospital.

*   *   *

When I returned to the apartment and Devin woke up, we ordered in a very late dinner.

After we ate, Devin was ready to go back to bed. In spite of the long nap he'd just enjoyed, he was exhausted from his lengthy ordeal, but a good night's sleep wasn't in the cards.

Once in bed, he began having extreme "creepy crawlies," that intense and persistent feeling of wanting to crawl out of your skin. Then phantom itching set in, and finally an agonizing rash crept up his trunk and face. It spread slowly, but by two in the morning, Devin was absolutely miserable and in tears.

We paged Dr. Chagnon, who sent us to the ER.

We were seen immediately, but the doctor couldn't figure out what was wrong. He gave Devin some heavy medication to help him sleep and stop the itching and told him he'd sleep soundly through the night even if these feelings continued.

If only he'd been right! Back at our apartment, Devin's insomnia was so extreme that in spite of being sedated, he couldn't drop off. I wrapped a blanket around him and held him in a sitting position in bed between my legs for the remainder of the night. For five and a half hours, I rocked him like a baby as he moaned and groaned in my arms.

At some point in the early morning, I broke down and called Sander, and it immediately became clear to him that Devin was experiencing severe withdrawal symptoms after suddenly stopping the opiates that had surged through his veins for the last 15 days.

In hindsight, I'm not sure why Dr. Chagnon and the ER doctor didn't recognize these symptoms. Perhaps it was because Devin was on opiates for much longer than the routine five to seven days and because he'd also received a multitude of other treatments at the same time his catheter was in place.

Under normal circumstances, medicines like oral ketamine, bisphosphonates, solumedral drips, and intrathecal catheters would be given to a patient one at a time spread over a longer period in order to determine the effect of each individual treatment.

Though not routine, Dr. Chagnon had felt we could safely hit Devin's pain from all angles during the brief period he was in her care, with the goal of eliminating his pain and not worrying so much about which treatment was responsible.

"The important thing now is to get rid of his pain," she'd explained.

Our son was going on a year of being dysfunctional and time was ticking, so we'd made the decision to go for it, but maybe the combination of all these treatments and medications was just too much for his sensitive system, or maybe these side effects weren't expected at all.

We decided it really didn't matter. What was important now was to somehow help Devin make it through this endless night, to endure yet one more bizarre and unexpected situation.

Finally, at around 7:30 in the morning, Devin collapsed and slept.

I hoped the worst was over, but he continued to experience severe insomnia for almost two weeks following discharge. His other symptoms slowly decreased, but it took almost two full weeks for them to disappear for good, too.

* * *

When we met with Dr. Chagnon a couple of days after Devin's discharge to discuss our next step, she mentioned the option of trying a spinal cord stimulator. She explained how this device is surgically implanted next to the spinal cord and provides a gentle, recurrent, pulsing sensation to the affected area through an electrical current. It had been successful for many of her patients, and if we could get Devin's pain under control for a period of time, maybe we could further reset his brain.

I didn't know what to say. We completely trusted Dr. Chagnon, but should we do this now, in Sonoma, or wait a couple of weeks until Devin wasn't so beat up and had more reserves?

Worn down, feeling as if I could no longer make a rational decision, I called my dad.

Without hesitation, he said, "Come home... now."

My relief was overwhelming. Devin was simply in no shape to go through another surgery so soon.

I was very grateful when Dr. Chagnon offered to help guide Devin's treatment from afar or consult with any doctors in our area. Her expertise, her persistence, and her belief in Devin, along with her certainty that we would find a cure, gave us the strength to keep going.

A full 22 days after our arrival, on August 28, my 46th birthday, we headed for home. This had been a much rougher experience than either of us had expected, and we didn't have much to say.

*   *   *

During our connection in Chicago, as we made our way to our gate, Devin and I both suddenly noticed that he was walking faster, with a significantly less noticeable limp.

"Mom, is it my imagination or am I actually walking faster?"

Devin was really excited, and so was I. To be walking better and faster this soon after lying in bed for 15 days surely meant we would see more progress as he continued to recover.

Sure enough, over the next several weeks, Devin began to walk without a limp for the first time in a year.

Meanwhile, in response to his decreased pain, we lowered his dose of Lyrica. By the end of our third week home, he was only taking 300 mg per day – half of what he'd taken at his peak. We were elated, for we knew this would reduce the side effects that made school so challenging.

Clearly, something had worked. California hadn't been easy, but now I was very grateful we had traveled the distance and Devin had endured the hell. We weren't where we wanted to be, but it was a start.

Chapter 6

The Emotional Roller Coaster Continues

September 15, 2008

Just came in from a long jog. It's a beautiful morning. The leaves are starting to turn and the bay is so blue and still. There isn't a single ripple on the water. I love when it's like this.

The run helped me sort out my thoughts. I need to be clearheaded when I go to the high school after lunch today to meet with Devin's teachers for his first official 504 meeting of the year. He's having a much harder time than we thought he would since we returned from California, and I need to get his teachers on board.

I was really hoping we would be done with all of this after how badly 8th grade went, but I guess not. He still can't think well. He still can't see well, and he's still in pain. I've got to help them understand this extremely complicated disease. How he has pain all the time, and how the effects from his pain meds make his vision impaired and learning very difficult for him. Most importantly, they've got to understand they need to make major modifications if he's going to be successful in their classes.

Sounds rather straightforward when I write it, but somehow it never is. They are going to have to be really understanding. I'm keeping my fingers crossed!

Our return from California at the end of August meant Devin was able to attend late registration before his first day of high school.

Thanks to the phone conferences I'd held in Sonoma with the 9th grade principal, the head high school principal, Devin's counselor, and the 504 coordinator, his new teachers were fully prepared for our high school freshman.

Initially, we had high hopes that the accommodations we'd set up might not be necessary. Devin was in better shape than last year, thanks to his diminished pain and reduced pain medication, but we soon realized his cognitive deficits remained overwhelming. He couldn't read, focus, process information, or remember what he'd learned. The only good news was that he didn't need a late pass this year. His gait was slow, but he no longer limped, and he could keep up with his friends.

As fall progressed, I spent many hours helping him prepare for quizzes and tests that in the past he would have easily and independently aced. Deep in a secret part of my heart, I wondered if his continuing cognitive difficulties might be a result of the oral ketamine he'd taken day after day in California. I knew Lyrica caused these problems too, but the phrase "no known long-term effects" I'd come across in numerous journal articles continued to worry me. Might there be long-term effects that simply hadn't yet been recognized?

As Sander and I commiserated about the reality of Devin's cognition, it occurred to my psychiatrist husband that Devin was having major attentional issues much like kids with ADD. He decided to put Devin through a specific computer test designed to look for attention deficits, and the results were eye opening. Not only was Devin extremely visually impaired with limited processing skills, the poor guy had absolutely no ability to focus.

Luckily, Sander had a few tricks up his sleeve and shared his ideas with Devin's prescribing physician. Devin had side effects to the first three trials of stimulants, but we finally found one that worked without causing additional problems. He still wasn't himself, but his processing abilities and his focus improved. Visual impairments aside, school became a little more manageable.

*   *   *

A high point in Devin's care at this time was working with Dr. Kersti Bruining. Dr. Bruining was the physician in our home town who we had carefully chosen to see Devin once we had returned from California. She was the neurologist who had performed a repeat EMG of his leg the previous winter, and had thoroughly impressed us with her comprehensive evaluation, which included listening carefully to both Devin and me.

I emphasize myself because when it comes to pain in kids, I found that many physicians are irritated when the parent tries to contribute information. They often think of us as meddling and seem to believe they will only get the truth by talking to the child.

I understand this to a degree, but the insight a mother or father can provide is crucial. If left solely to the child, certain key aspects would be overlooked. This was certainly the case with Devin. He wasn't thinking clearly most of the time because of his pain medication and would have left gaping holes in his history.

Happily, Dr. Bruining respected both Devin's and my input. We knew immediately that she cared about and believed in Devin. She didn't have a lot of experience with CRPS, but we trusted that she would consult with Dr. Chagnon in California and search for answers to the best of her ability, and she did.

Interestingly, while she was trying to do the EMG at that first appointment in February, Devin's right leg had been so cold she couldn't get an accurate result. She'd had to stop the test and get a heating pad to see if she could normalize the temperature. She couldn't, so she'd done the EMG as best she could. Her documentation of the temperature difference came in handy while seeing other physicians later on, especially if Devin's leg wasn't showing temperature changes that particular day.

We didn't have this documentation with us at our meeting with the Wisconsin doctor, but we applied the maxim "Live and learn" and made sure we had it with us at all subsequent doctor's appointments.

*   *   *

During Dr. Bruining's initial phone consultation with Dr. Chagnon, she learned about the recommendation for Devin to receive a spinal cord stimulator. Fully recovered from his recent ICU experience, yet still riddled with the pain of CRPS, Devin was now interested and ready to try out this promising new technology.

A physician in our hometown had just received a spinal cord stimulator to treat his own CRPS. He had great results, and recommended we see a specialist at the University of Michigan who did training for the company that supplies stimulators to doctors all around the country.

This specialist was one of the top neurosurgeons in the region. He wasn't an expert on CRPS, but that didn't matter. We didn't need advice on CRPS or a conferring of diagnosis; we just wanted his advice on spinal cord stimulators and hopefully his approval to schedule Devin for a trial.

We couldn't get in until late November, but our son Ethan, now a senior in high school, had just learned he'd been accepted to the University of Michigan. We decided to make a trip out of it and tour the campus while we were there.

To our dismay, after waiting two months for this appointment, the specialist briskly entered the examining room, performed a quick evaluation lasting all of five minutes, then spent three more minutes talking to Devin before concluding he didn't have CRPS. He explained that Devin would have to be much more disabled and his leg would have to be bright red, cold, and swollen for this diagnosis to be made.

Before my very eyes, Devin's face turned grey.

The doctor hadn't read any of Devin's records, so Sander and I tried to show him the documentation of the temperature difference from Dr. Bruining. We tried to tell him about Devin's three-week stay in California where his diagnosis had already been made. We tried to tell him we weren't there for his opinion about Devin's diagnosis, just for advice on a stimulator, but he'd run out of time and the appointment was over.

We were stunned, furious, and demoralized. We had traveled all the way to Ann Arbor, an eight-hour round trip, for eight minutes of horrible advice that set us back, psychologically at least, to our nightmare the previous February in Wisconsin.

At that moment, in spite of coming from a huge family of physicians including my husband, my father, my sister, my brother, many of my uncles, my father-in-law, two sisters-in law, a brother-in-law, and a number of uncles and cousins, I lost the deep and enduring faith I have always had in physicians.

Nonetheless, for Devin's sake, we tried not to harbor too much on this negative experience. Instead, we dismissed this physician as he'd dismissed us and called our trip to Ann Arbor successful for having toured U of M's campus. We also decided to have a local anesthesiologist, an acquaintance of ours from our hometown, evaluate and perform the spinal cord stimulator trial.

Dr. Richard Burke had been following Devin's case all along because his son and Ethan are good buddies. He'd told Ethan many times to have us call him if we were interested in a spinal cord stimulator because he performed this surgery almost daily.

After he saw Devin and evaluated him as appropriate for a trial, he scheduled him for surgery at our local hospital's pain center the following week.

Step one required implanting a spinal cord stimulator with the main lead remaining external so Devin could adjust the frequency and wave lengths himself to see if he could find a comfortable setting. If the trial was successful, the lead would be surgically implanted and controlled by a wireless remote.

The initial surgery was a bit more than we expected and the implant was very uncomfortable. Over the next two days, Devin noticed a 20% or so decrease in his pain after experimenting with the settings, but his relief didn't improve any further. This meant the trial was a failure. To be considered a success, patients need to feel at least 50% pain relief.

Accordingly, we had the spinal cord stimulator removed and checked it off our list. Devin missed a couple days of school and experienced a few days of additional discomfort, but it was worth a try, and now we could turn our attention to addressing a rather big hurdle at school.

* * *

In addition to Devin's other accommodations, he was scheduled to have a free hour each trimester during his freshman year. He desperately needed this extra time, since simply reading his large print worksheets took him three times as long as the other kids.

The problem was, giving him this extra hour meant he was going to be one and a half credits behind his classmates at the end of his 9th grade year. If, heaven forbid, he required a partial schedule throughout his four years of high school, it was going to take some creative scheduling for him to earn enough credits to graduate with his classmates.

Our research on 504 programming for students with CRPS had already helped us inform teachers about 504 regulations and typical learning issues that occur with CRPS. One specific recommendation, giving gym credit to kids involved in on-going extensive physical therapy services, caught our attention.

To us, this made intuitive sense. Kids like Devin were already doing a tremendous amount of physical therapy and exercise on a daily basis, well above the hours necessary for gym credit. This would be a way for them to get credit that would otherwise be hard to earn since most of them were on a partial schedule throughout high school due to their limitations from medications and pain.

Armed with this information, midway through his freshman year of high school, I decided to present Devin's case to the administration and request that he receive gym credit for his therapy in lieu of taking a gym class.

We spoke to the 504 coordinator, the 9th grade principal, and the school nurse. All three agreed this was a "no brainer," but told me I must take this request to the head principal, who was strongly opposed to the idea and wanted to speak to me in person.

I wasn't worried. To date, everyone I had spoken to was in our corner. Prudently, I prepared the information I would need if the principal wasn't responsive, but I had faith that common sense would save the day.

A few days before our meeting on an unseasonably cold and snowy December morning, I drove to the school and gave the principal a letter explaining Devin's condition and history as well as information about CRPS and the 504 program recommendations on providing gym credit for students with CRPS. I expected his resistance came from a lack of knowledge about this disease, and I fully expected that once he saw the recommendations for 504 programming in black and white, he would change his mind.

Today, I just shake my head at my own naiveté. I'd heard rumors the principal was extremely rigid. I'd heard he was recruited solely to whip the high school into shape. I'd heard his job was to eliminate troubled kids, troubled teachers, bad rules, and bad precedents, and then be on his merry way.

What's more, Ethan had told me many tales about just how much and why he was disliked by the student body, but I'd stubbornly chosen to give the principal the benefit of the doubt. On more than one occasion, I'd told my firstborn the principal simply couldn't be that bad; he just had a hard job to do, and that's why he wasn't the most popular guy on the block.

The day of our appointment, I walked into the principal's office feeling confident, but it only took me a moment to see that I was up against someone with little human compassion and extreme rigidity issues. He was smug and aloof, and my confidence quickly dissipated.

I spoke briefly about Devin's history, and a small grin broke out on his face as if he knew something I did not. A bit bewildered, I explained the rationale for our request to give gym credit to Devin.

When I finished, he said, "You know, Wendy, the school will take care of Devin. I don't know why you're so worried. I don't see why you have Devin on a 504 plan in the first place. It's an archaic 1970's law that means nothing."

I was utterly bemused. First of all, what did he mean, "The school will take care of Devin"? Second of all, was I hearing what I thought I was hearing? That the head principal of the high school didn't agree with 504 plans?

I carefully replied that the 504 plan was extremely helpful for Devin. I explained that it provided us with a 504 coordinator who helped us coordinate a plan with all of Devin's teachers. I explained that it allowed us to have regular meetings so we could keep them abreast of Devin's disability and any changes in his situation. I explained that the teachers were always grateful to be kept up to date, and how thankful we were to know we were all on the same page. Then I asked why he didn't think Devin needed a 504 plan.

"People on a 504 plan don't have confidence that the school and teachers will take care of their child," he promptly replied. "This high school takes care of its students, and we don't need a silly plan to get us to do so."

"How do you plan to 'take care of Devin'?" I asked.

He replied, "If Devin can't complete his gym requirement by his senior year, it will be waived."

I told him I appreciated this, but that I was already familiar with this policy. Of course gym would be waived for a kid like Devin.

"What I'm asking for," I earnestly explained, "is credit for Devin's intense physical therapy and exercise program that I provided to you in detail prior to this meeting."

I explained again that Devin was already going to be one and a half credits behind his peers at the end of the year and very possibly many more credits behind by the end of high school. I showed him the pamphlet I had downloaded that clearly spelled out these 504 recommendations, which I was increasingly certain he hadn't read.

When he continued to wear that annoying, smug smirk, I asked why he was opposed to providing gym credit for a boy in Devin's unique situation.

"I can't start a precedent," he replied matter-of-factly. "I am working hard to take away poor precedents that have been set up, and I refuse to start this one. Do you think every student who has a broken leg or a sore arm should get credit for their gym?"

In a shaky voice, I told him that Devin's illness was an ongoing chronic condition that wouldn't heal like a broken bone. It affected all parts of his learning and his ability to take on a full schedule and couldn't be compared with a broken bone. I repeated that this disability required special individualized services. Thus, Devin was not to be looked at as a precedent but rather a unique situation. Handling certain medical situations and disabilities with special programming did not set a precedent, I explained, because these students were labeled as 504 students with very specific needs, which in and of itself explained the need for 504 plans.

To this impassioned speech, he replied that he'd just remembered he'd written on Devin's school plan that if by graduation he hadn't completed his gym credits, they were to be given to him at that point.

I shook my head. He might be retired or gone by then, which would allow any other administrator to potentially misinterpret this request. If they refused, it would be too late to do anything about it. I emphasized this was something we needed to resolve *now*.

My suspicions raised, I asked to see this written documentation.

The principal fumbled for a moment, then got onto his computer and found a file on Devin.

Over his shoulder, I silently read through it. Not surprisingly, nothing was written about Devin being allowed to receive gym credit at the time of graduation, only that he could have gym waived if need be.

"This information isn't written in Devin's file," I quietly told the principal. "Why did you tell me it was?"

He was embarrassed, quickly turned off his computer, and abruptly changed the subject.

Sternly, he told me that in his opinion, Ethan should feel horrible about what he'd done to his brother, but he didn't appear to care about Devin and was insensitive to others as well. What's more, the principal emphasized, Ethan was overly active and could injure Devin again.

I knew this paragon of virtue had recently reprimanded Ethan at a football game for being too rowdy. I had no issue with that, and there was no need to discuss it. The issue was how inappropriate it was for him to bring Ethan up at this time and in this way.

In retrospect, I realize the principal was trying to distract me from having caught him in a lie, but at that moment, hearing him criticize Ethan caused me to crumble. Ethan felt terrible that his brother's life had changed, that all our lives had changed. He felt terrible that he'd been involved.

I felt so vulnerable, so frustrated, and so bewildered that anyone in this man's position could be such a bully that I began to cry. I tried in vain not to, but tears coursed down my cheeks and I had to choke back sobs.

I got up to leave, but the principal told me he didn't want me to go because people would see me crying and wonder what he'd done.

He actually got up from his desk and blocked the door, but I asked him to move and I quickly left.

As soon as I reached the safety of my car, I called Sander, crying uncontrollably.

When I told him what happened, he reminded me this was exactly why we have 504 plans: to protect students with disabilities – legally if necessary – from schools that may not be willing to provide an educational setting that will work with them.

After talking it through, we agreed to begin the appeals process and file a motion for a hearing with the school system. We had prepared the necessary paperwork to do this; I just hadn't believed anyone could be so uncaring and manipulative. I hadn't believed I would need to force the issue.

When Sander and I hung up, I was so angry I drove straight to the administration building and talked with the district's 504 coordinator. To my surprise, she'd never before been confronted with a 504 issue.

I told her what had happened and explained that if I put my request for a hearing into writing, the school had 15 days to respond. I handed her this information to review. I also had a scribbled letter requesting a hearing, written just moments before in the car, and I gave that to her as well.

She looked a little stunned. She said she didn't even know what to do with the information, but she would give it to the assistant superintendent and have her contact us with next steps.

Later that afternoon, I received a phone call from the assistant superintendent. She knows Sander well because he does numerous gratis lectures for the school system, the community, and the teachers. She had me briefly go over our original request and the circumstances leading to our request for a hearing and then confided that nobody to date had requested, much less gone, to hearing. She assured me the last thing the school wanted was to go to hearing for political and financial reasons. She asked, if she could resolve this with the head principal, would we be willing to remove the request for a hearing?

"Of course," was my response. Resolution was all we'd ever wanted. I was even ready to tuck my tail between my legs and confess to Ethan that he'd been absolutely right about the principal. I wasn't a member of the student body, but I despised him too!

* * *

Immediately following winter break, I received a call from the 9th grade principal letting me know Devin could receive full gym credit if he kept a detailed log of his physical therapy and exercise program and if there were ongoing letters from his physical therapist.

With a deep sigh, I thanked him and told him this was exactly what we had hoped for. I would much rather work amiably with people than play hardball, but when you are taking care of a chronically ill child, you become extremely strong, even if you break down and cry when confronted by those who are unsympathetic and despicable. Your protective instincts set in and you know you can't let anything stop you from doing what is right for your child. You can't worry about impending conflict or what other people who don't fully understand the situation will think. For the sake of your child, for the love of your child, you just have to trust your instincts and do the right thing.

Chapter 7

Desperate Times Call for Desperate Measures

December 12, 2008

It's Devin's 15th birthday! What a fun day! I spent the morning at the elementary school watching Taylor play the lead female role in her 5th grade science musical. Something about rocks and geology...Anyway, it was very cute and she was great! It's these little things that keep me going these days.

I spent the rest of the day running around town trying to make Devin's birthday really special. I got his favorite chocolate cream pie and lots of little gifts and CD's and invited his friends over for dinner and presents. I spoil him a lot these days even when it's not his birthday. It's just that he's so sweet and has been through, and is still going through, way too much for a kid his age. No one should have to go through this nightmare. I'm going to take any opportunity I can to make his day a little brighter. I can't take away his pain, but at least I can do this.

I have to remember later to ask him what he's been researching on the internet about CRPS. He's been on the computer a lot and mentioned he found something interesting?

Dr. Chagnon had seen full recovery from CRPS in teens even 18 months after the original injury. We were rapidly approaching this date, and Devin was understandably frustrated. Although his pain was under better control after his time in California, it was still significant and constant. The slightest touch to his leg made him scream, and minor bumps still rendered him dysfunctional. Very resourceful throughout this whole experience in spite of his cognitive challenges and vision problems, he was doing his own research on CRPS and the different types of treatment options.

After surfing the internet persistently, he became very excited about one particular approach that used low-dose intravenous ketamine, not the oral ketamine he'd had in California, as an infusion for five days.

As we'd learned during our time in California, ketamine acts as a NMDA receptor block, preventing glutamate from binding to this receptor within the dorsal horn of the spinal cord. By blocking this receptor, it prevents the transfer of pain signals between the second order neuron within the spinal cord and the brain.

The flipside to this, in patients with CRPS, is a constant and prolonged release of glutamate in this area of the spinal cord that can lead to a process known as central sensitization – a phenomenon that maintains a permanent state of hyperactivity and pain perception within the central nervous system.

Intravenous ketamine's ability to inhibit these receptors, Devin learned, has been known to reverse the effects of central sensitization and has been very effective for many people suffering from CRPS. For most individuals, it has completely taken away their pain and for a lesser few has provided partial pain benefits.

Low-dose IV ketamine infusions aren't a cure – the pain relief often wears off anywhere from two weeks to two years after being administered – but when given a second time, this treatment is typically more effective and lasts longer.

Even though he knew ketamine couldn't be considered the final answer, Devin hoped it might break the pain cycle long enough to provide much needed relief and allow him to function at a higher level, which could lead to better rehabilitation and a more permanent decrease in his pain. The main difference, he learned, between the oral ketamine he'd tried in California and the IV ketamine approach was the blood concentration level of the drug. When given intravenously, the concentration was much higher and thus more effective.

In response to Devin's enthusiasm, Sander and I reluctantly began our own additional research on ketamine. We found three ways of using it to treat pain besides taking it orally: the five-day low-dose IV ketamine infusion which Devin had discovered, an outpatient IV ketamine infusion given to the patient for four to six hours at a time spread over two weeks to many months, and a non-FDA-approved five-day ketamine coma only offered in Mexico and Germany. We also discovered a three-day outpatient "close to coma" ketamine version currently being researched in Florida.

The benefits of the ketamine-induced coma were discovered accidentally when a patient from Germany with a pre-existing case of CRPS suffered severe trauma from a car accident. She was put into an induced coma in order to protect her brain, and when she awakened, her chronic pain was completely gone.

Since this discovery, dozens of patients have been treated with this aggressive, controversial technique in Germany as well as Mexico. Half have come out of the coma state completely cured, with no pain and no return of symptoms. The remaining patients either have return of symptoms, partial pain relief, or no results at all.

As exciting as these results are, the coma is extreme, requires intubation, and comes with substantial risks. Some patients, after awakening from the coma, are extremely disoriented, have loss of memory and motor function, and may require weeks or months of cognitive and physical rehabilitation solely to recover from the effects of the coma.

While all research indicates it should only be considered as a last resort, some professionals call the "ketamine coma" the only lasting cure for CRPS. It is typically reserved for patients who have tried every other approach over many years with no success and who have become completely incapacitated, dysfunctional, and desperate.

* * *

Back on the home front, Devin asked us to look further into the five-day low-dose "awake" ketamine infusion. He was understandably fearful of the coma and optimistically believed that the "awake" version, which held much less risk, could eliminate his pain for good.

Sander and I thought we would never consider ketamine again after watching Devin suffer its effects in California. I wasn't the least bit interested in having this drug surging through my son's body 24 hours a day for five to seven days. However, seeing as the spinal cord stimulator hadn't worked and we'd hit another road block, we unenthusiastically told Devin we'd look into it.

We did a literature search through the hospital, researched every possible article on the internet, and located each physician in the United States who performed this procedure. Sander started making phone calls, and after a lengthy discussion with a physician routinely using ketamine to treat patients with CRPS, he began to feel much more comfortable with the idea.

This doctor believed low-dose ketamine was very safe. He emphasized that if the protocol was followed correctly and appropriate precautions were taken, the "awake" version held minimal risks. Likewise, he didn't believe there were any long-term problems associated with it. Nonetheless, he told Sander that patients are typically monitored in an intensive care unit since blood levels, liver functions, and levels of consciousness need to be closely monitored.

Sander located two additional physicians both on the cutting edge of using ketamine and passed all three names on to Dr. Bruining. Like Devin, we were becoming very excited about the possibilities of ketamine, and it was our growing hope that she would be willing to help us get a team of physicians together to perform this protocol right here at our local hospital.

We were asking a lot of Dr. Bruining – no one in our small town had used or possibly even heard of using ketamine in this way – but after doing her own research, she also became energized about the possibilities.

What Dr. Bruining did next was truly incredible. She somehow managed to gather a group of physicians at our local hospital including a pediatrician, an intensivist, an anesthesiologist, and a pharmacist. Once they signed on, she directed this treatment approach through the hospital review committee as well as our insurance company.

Having the hospital consent was a huge hurdle, but getting our insurance company to preauthorize this treatment was unheard of. Until now, nobody in the country had been able to get reimbursement for ketamine as a treatment for CRPS. How she managed this miracle, I don't know. What I do know is that she put in many, many hours to make this happen for Devin, and to say we are grateful is woefully inadequate. The ketamine infusion was our current best hope, and if it hadn't materialized at our local hospital, we would have been forced to approach one of the other doctors in the United States who used low-dose IV ketamine for CRPS and endure the typical year-long waiting list. While Devin waited for treatment, time would have continued slipping away.

* * *

Devin was scheduled to be admitted to the ICU during the first week of Christmas break. As the date approached, I have to admit I grew increasingly scared. Dr. Bruining had selected a well-published approach used by one of the leading physicians in the country, but I couldn't help but wonder if we should be doing this at a hospital with experienced physicians and staff. Was our ICU capable of handling this? My husband and Dr. Bruining both felt confident, so I chose to be as well, at least on the surface.

We admitted Devin on a Monday, and Sander and I took turns staying with him around the clock. After blood work, heart monitor hook-ups, and insertion of the IV, they began the infusion. The goal was to have Devin receive 40 mg/hour of ketamine for five full days. The protocol suggested waiting for the pain to either be at 0 out of

10 on the pain scale or plateau at its lowest level for 48 hours before stopping the IV.

The first evening was uneventful, and Devin felt little effect from the ketamine, most likely because the infusion rate was being brought up so slowly.

By early morning, as the rate increased, Devin started to feel the effects much more powerfully. Sander had spent the night, and by the time I arrived at 7:00 a.m. and Sander left for work, Devin was beginning to have a rough time.

Soon, he was experiencing strong hallucinations and the same facial paralysis and loss of coordination I had seen in California. On top of this, he began to vomit, and I mean a lot!

We tried different medications to calm the nausea. Ativan finally seemed to help, but Devin still continued to vomit intermittently throughout the day. He seemed extremely "drugged out" and had a hard time talking or communicating. Between his hallucinations, lack of coordination, anxiety, vomiting, and overall deteriorating mental state, this was quite a scary situation, and I was extremely worried. Adding to my discomfort was the fact that we had no idea what we were in for. This was day one, and we were going to do this for five full days?

By the end of the first day, we realized Devin had not urinated, so a catheter was placed. He also had been unable to eat. We feared that if he were in this state for the full five days, we might need to get him nutrition via a different route. The IV team came and decided to place a PICC line in his right arm so that both nutrition and medication could be administered at the same time.

I had never seen this done before, and while I'm told it's usually a straightforward procedure, it took the IV team an inordinate amount of time to place the catheter because Devin's veins kept collapsing. Even in his semi-conscious state, I noticed tears in his eyes as I held his hand during this exceptionally long and uncomfortable procedure.

It was heart-wrenching to watch him go through this, and I wondered how much more he could take before he decided it was easier to live with his unremitting, debilitating pain than undergo such procedures. I remained calm and confident on the outside, but inside I was completely torn up. This situation felt particularly unbearable, as I didn't know what was in store for him over the next few days.

I didn't sleep a wink that night, between trying to get comfortable on the hospital chair-bed, worrying about Devin, the loud alarms that went off repetitively each time an IV was close to empty or became kinked, and the regular visits from the nurse. Devin was so out of it that, hour after hour, the nurse resorted to screaming at him to get him alert to check his level of consciousness.

After a seemingly endless night, Devin slowly roused. As the morning went on, he appeared to be doing a bit better. He was still inebriated and hallucinating, but he could now communicate about what he was experiencing. His pain stubbornly remained at 6 ½ for most of the day, but around 5:00 p.m., he said his leg was starting to feel better. When he rated it a 5 ½, I couldn't believe it. The ketamine was starting to work!

By the next day, he was no longer nauseated, just really goofy. He was seeing hallucinations that he found funny and was extremely verbal. He even believed he had a nurse who didn't exist whom he affectionately named Joe. Everything was super colorful, in duplicate, and zooming by. At one point, I walked to the other side of the room and he yelled, "Whoa! Slow down. How did you get there so fast? You're like lightening!"

Devin was comfortable like this, and he remained in this condition for the rest of his hospitalization. I must confess, his new state of mind provided some much-needed comic relief. His friends, his brother, and his brother's friends had a ball with him, and Devin certainly enjoyed their company.

Once Devin was in this stable condition, Taylor came to visit each day with either Sander or me. On her first visit, she brought him a bright red "silly man" squeeze ball he fondly named "K." His new friend "K" became his obsession for the remainder of his stay.

To our joy, his pain kept decreasing. Each day, he was down another half point or so. Even better, as his pain decreased, Dr. Bruining began to wean him off his medication.

Based on her research and that of Devin's other doctors, we mutually agreed to keep him in the ICU on ketamine past the typical five days since his pain hadn't yet stopped going down.

By day six, the effects of the ketamine appeared to be slowing. Devin's pain was now at a 2 ½, and he was no longer taking *any* of the medication that had been causing such havoc in his life.

We waited two more days as the protocol suggested to be sure he had plateaued. Once we were satisfied, we weaned him from the ketamine and went home.

As we walked out of the hospital that snowy afternoon with Christmas lights and holiday spirit surrounding us, we could already tell we had our son back. The hallucinations and goofy effects of the ketamine had disappeared, and that wonderful content smile of Devin's we hadn't seen in so long was back.

He immediately started lovingly teasing his little sister and giving his dad a hard time about the silly shirt he was wearing. The stress that had been etched on Devin's adolescent face for so many months was gone, and his sarcasm and good humor had returned in full force.

The first thing he did when we got home was take a shower. After eight days of going without, this wasn't a surprise, but what he did next simply amazed us.

He picked up a book. Just like that, his vision had returned. After 14 months of not being able to read, he picked up a book and read... easily! Not only that, he understood and remembered what he read.

Later that night, he even opened his history textbook in order to catch up on some work he'd missed before Christmas break.

Still taking it all in, I asked if he needed me to go over the worksheet with him.

His response was, "I'm fine, Mom."

I said, "What do you mean, you're 'fine'?"

He smiled. "I read the chapter and I can do the worksheet on my own. I remember what I read and it makes perfect sense to me."

Blown away, I walked into the kitchen in shock. He wasn't quite at 0 on the pain scale, but the ketamine infusion had obviously worked.

The next few weeks were amazing. First of all, Devin was almost pain free for the first time in 15 months. Second, he jumped back into school as if he'd never skipped a beat. He studied independently, received A's on his tests and assignments, and took full initiative for his work. He was thinking like the quick, bright young man he'd always been. To see him so happy, playing the piano, and having so much fun with his friends seemed a miracle. He still couldn't run, but he was walking faster and keeping up.

Oh yes, and you could also touch his leg. You could even bump hard into his leg! Maggie jumped onto his lap one night and pawed his right leg, and Devin didn't react at all. He didn't hurt. We laughed for joy to see him gently roughhousing with his dog as in days past rather than avoiding her for fear she'd inadvertently hurt him.

This was a sweet, sweet time. All our lives reverted to normal. With Devin functioning beautifully at school, I was able to devote myself once again to the normal tasks of a busy mom who had been neglecting her home and to some degree her husband and other children a little too long.

Sander, Ethan, and Taylor reveled in regular home-cooked meals and dependably clean laundry, and I reveled in being able to focus on their lives, interests, and activities. Devin was thriving, and I was no longer unnaturally preoccupied with him.

I felt like we had the world by the tail.

*   *   *

About three and a half weeks after his release from the hospital, Devin sat uncharacteristically still one evening, a serious look on his face.

That terrible and all-too-familiar feeling of heaviness slowly began to consume my body. I took a long deep breath before pressing him, but I already knew what he was going to say. I had seen this expression on his face too many times before.

Devin softly said, "Mom, I think my pain is starting to come back."

Over the next few days, his pain crept up to a 4. The following week, it was closer to a 6 ½ and he missed two days of school. By the next week, it had skyrocketed back to a 9. With the effects of the ketamine worn off and no medications to control the pain, Devin, bedridden, missed the entire next week of school.

We struggled with what to do. With Dr. Bruining's support, we decided to re-administer the ketamine infusion ASAP. We were determined to do everything possible to avoid putting him back on those debilitating pain medicines. Our son's innate ability to learn had returned, and we couldn't bear to give him medications that would compromise it.

According to the material we read, the second round of ketamine would work much faster, last much longer, and possibly bring the pain to a lower level.

We had been prepared to schedule a second infusion at some point in the spring anyway, we consoled ourselves; we were just scheduling it much sooner than planned.

Luckily, we were able to get hospital and insurance approval for that Friday, and we braced ourselves for round two.

Chapter 8

An Unexpected Bombshell

February 3, 2009

I feel sick. I've been feeling this way for six days now. I literally feel like I've been slugged in the stomach multiple times. My insides actually feel bruised. I feel so heavy and so weighed down, I almost can't move. I know this is emotional and I know that I have no time to indulge in this feeling. Most importantly, I know I can't let Devin sense how I feel.

He somehow has to be confident that Sander and I are endlessly strong, optimistic, and in control and that we will make him better and make his pain go away. Our confidence when we tell him we will figure this out soon has somehow kept him going since his pain came back so fiercely last week. I see it in his eyes when we talk to him. Right now, Devin is relying on our strength.

How brutal it must have been to briefly have his life back and then for it to cruelly be ripped away. It doesn't make any sense! He just wants his life back! Is that too much to ask?

For the love of god….He just wants to be a teenager…He just wants to be happy! I hope with all my heart that this next round of ketamine will work…that it will <u>last</u>!

After warm welcomes from the friendly staff in the ICU, Devin was re-admitted. He unpacked his things in the same spacious room as before, the one with the attractive view of the parking lot, and after his blood was redrawn and his vitals re-taken, he was hooked back up to the magical ketamine.

We were prepared for a bad first 24 hours like last time and scheduled our round-the-clock shifts accordingly, but this time, the effects from the drug were much less severe, almost nonexistent. Devin had no hallucinations, no nausea, and remained fairly lucid throughout the seven days of his treatment. The pharmacist assured us that even with the lack of inebriation, the ketamine should do its thing just as effectively.

While this was good news in and of itself, we were a little sobered to think Devin's brain had become accustomed to the ketamine. Was it possible our child had so much ketamine pumping through him that he was becoming tolerant to this heavy street drug?

Two days went by, then three, before Devin finally started to feel some pain relief. By day five, his pain had dropped to about a 5. Initially, we were pleased. Devin could function again. We waited another day and a half, but nothing more happened. The pain would budge no more, and we became very discouraged. His response was supposed to be better this time; his pain was supposed to bottom out closer to zero. What had happened?

Dr. Bruining contacted the doctor whose ketamine protocol we were following. He was more than happy to consult, and he recommended we try to augment the ketamine by having Devin receive a few different spinal treatments to the area of his original injury. These included a radiofrequency ablation, or RFA (a medical procedure in which a portion of the electrical conduction system of a tissue is destroyed using a high frequency alternating current), steroid injections to further decrease inflammation, and Botox injections to decrease potential muscle spasms that could be aggravating the original injury site.

These treatments needed to be administered at the hospital's outpatient surgical pain clinic a few miles from the hospital. This meant Devin and I would have to drive there, and Devin would receive these procedures as an out-patient before returning to the ICU to be re-hooked up to the ketamine.

We never mentioned it to his nurse, but on our way to the pain center the next morning, we snuck to the home of a friend who lived near the hospital so Devin could take a quick shower. This was the high point of the week for him.

All fresh and clean, Devin entered the pain center with a positive attitude, ready to endure whatever they threw at him. He was accustomed to being poked and prodded, and very little ruffled his feathers at this point. He never complained about the need for these procedures or worried that they'd hurt. He just casually talked and joked about being a human pincushion as he waited to be wheeled into the operating room.

The doctor treating Devin was Dr. Burke, the same physician who'd done the trial spinal cord stimulator. Devin greeted him with a smile on his face, comfortable in his care.

The radiofrequency ablation was to be performed three times. Accordingly, an electrode attached to a radiofrequency machine was placed in Devin's spine and the radiofrequency machine was slowly turned up until it provided a strong vibrating sensation to his right leg for two minutes.

The first round seemed to go well.

The second time around, the technician turned the knob quite far and Devin's leg began to spasm hard. He looked extremely uncomfortable and grimaced in pain, his face turning as white as a ghost, but he was willing to continue after the frequency was lowered to a tolerable level.

Immediately following the third trial, Dr. Burke injected steroid to the site as recommended. Dr. Bruining would give Devin the Botox injections once he was comfortably resituated back at the hospital.

Devin remained extremely compliant, but as he was brought to recovery, I noticed tears streaming down his face. He was obviously in terrible pain, and when I questioned him, he told me he was at a 9 or higher. Before this procedure, his pain had been at a 5.

Completely unsure of myself, I told him this was probably normal after the procedure he'd just received and that it would begin to resolve soon. I had no idea if this was true, but it was definitely more productive to try to be positive and hopeful than to embrace the worst.

With Devin in agony, we left the pain center and drove back to the hospital. As I wheeled him back up to the ICU, for the first time in the course of nearly a year and a half of treatment, he began to protest. Quite simply, he'd had it. He didn't understand why we had to come back to the hospital, why he had to be re-connected to the ketamine, and why we'd done these "stupid procedures." He just wanted to go home and curl up on his bed.

*   *   *

Sander joined us at about 6:30 that evening. Although I'd prepared him ahead of time, he was quite shaken to see Devin so agitated, so teary, and in such acute pain.

Dr. Bruining came in around 8:00 p.m. She tried to comfort Devin by telling him she felt hopeful the pain was from these new procedures and that it would soon begin to subside. She explained that he must stay in the ICU for a few more days to see if the combination of the new procedures along with the ketamine would drop his pain below the 5 he'd experienced earlier today. As she was trying to console him, she instinctively patted him on the leg closest to her.

As luck would have it, it was Devin's right leg, and he sent up such a howl I thought he'd awaken the entire hospital and bring on the police. I had never seen him in such a heightened state of pain; I had never seen him cry like this.

Balling, he begged poor remorseful Dr. Bruining to let him go home, but she couldn't discharge him in such acute pain. What's more, she was determined to keep him at least two more days with the ketamine back on board.

In desperation, Sander, Dr. Bruining, and I discussed a new

plan that included getting him back on pain medication. He simply couldn't go on like this, and we decided to try new medications that hopefully wouldn't interfere with his vision or thinking.

Our plan in place, we briefly walked out of the room together. Dr. Bruining remained calm and encouraging, but I had never felt so discouraged. This was easily Devin's lowest moment since this whole ordeal began, and I believe it was mine as well. Until now, when something hadn't worked or his pain returned, we had optimistically moved on to the next approach.

This time, the dangerous ketamine coma aside, there was nothing left to try. We had researched ourselves silly and taken extreme measures, and we were in worse shape now than ever before. For the first time, I entertained the thought that Devin might have to live with this syndrome, with this kind of pain, for the rest of his life.

I can't even begin to explain how I felt at this moment. The realization that my 15-year-old might have to endure this type of suffering for the rest of his life caused such sadness. I was paralyzed by an indescribable level of emotion. Once again, I wondered how much longer he could tolerate it. How much longer could I tolerate watching him go through this?

In the hallway, Sander and I did our best to console each other and gather strength before entering the room again to be with Devin. As devastated as we were, I knew we couldn't let him see the depth of our fear or despair. Though mature beyond his years, he was still a child, and he would take our lead, for better or worse. Somehow, it had to be for better.

*   *   *

Newly resolved to stay strong for Devin's sake, we walked back into his room, prepared for the worst.

Devin had wiped away his tears and wanted to talk with us.

This was obviously something big, but we had no idea what he was about to say. I must admit, absolutely nothing could have prepared us for what was coming.

Over the last year and a half, Devin had openly communicated with us about his pain and how he was coping. Always optimistic, he had continued to see each day as the day we might discover a new treatment that could beat his disease. Apparently, his present state of pain was too much for him.

In one of the most intense discussions we've ever had with our son, Devin solemnly informed us that his suffering had become unbearable and that he could no longer endure it day in and day out. He told us we could never understand what living with this type of chronic pain was like and that he was at his wit's end trying to find some way to control it.

It was true; Devin had spent almost as much time as Sander and I on the internet looking for an answer and trying to understand CRPS. What we didn't know was that he'd also been doing a lot of research on medical marijuana, which had just become legalized in the state of Michigan in November.

Devin took a deep breath and quietly informed us that in the last several months, he'd tried marijuana a couple of times when his pain was really bad and that it had provided the best pain control of any medication he'd been on.

Sander and I were speechless, but Devin had more to say. He explained that he'd only tried it for this purpose and he had no interest in using it recreationally, but he felt it was time to begin using it regularly to control his pain.

We were still dumbstruck, so he reminded us that he'd been very patient and willing to go through all sorts of treatments. He told us he had full confidence in us and Dr. Bruining, but nothing was working. If he was going to have to live like this for the rest of his life, he would need to use cannabis to get through it.

As politely as possible and without any drama whatsoever, he informed us that he wanted us to help him become licensed to use medical marijuana. He also told us that if we didn't help him, he would continue to seek it out on his own when he felt he really needed a break from the pain.

The buzzing in my ears made me so disoriented, I wondered if I'd heard him correctly. My sweet, clean-cut, 15-year-old son was asking permission to use medical marijuana? He was telling us that even if we said no, he would use it without our knowing in order to relieve his pain? He hoped we would help him, but if not, at least he wanted to be honest?

My mouth must have been hanging open. In November, just a few short months ago, I'd voted against the legalization of medical marijuana. I knew it could be an issue for my son at some point in the future, and I didn't want him to see it as a form of palliative care, much less legal palliative care.

I couldn't help but feel marijuana use could potentially have significant social consequences. How would other kids, parents, teachers, and family members view Devin if he were using marijuana on a regular basis to control his pain? More importantly, I was concerned about the harmful long-term effects regular cannabis use could have on his still developing brain.

At the same time, if it weren't for Devin, I knew I probably would have voted "yes" on this proposal. If marijuana helps cancer victims or others with intractable pain go on living or manage their otherwise uncontrollable pain, I believe it should be legalized.

I'm pretty sure the color completely drained from my face when Devin laid this bombshell at our feet, but after a very deep breath, both Sander and I responded heroically. I say "heroically" because, although cool and collected on the outside, I wanted to explode on the inside. We didn't want Devin to feel he'd made a mistake confiding in us. We felt fortunate he'd told us. Yet we both realized we had a sticky situation on our hands.

If we'd said, "Are you crazy? Absolutely not!" our son would most likely buy marijuana from some drug dealer on the street and use it behind our backs. If we agreed to help him become legalized, we would get ourselves in a position that could be hard to reverse.

Though this wasn't Devin's intention, we were being backed into a corner.

We calmly asked Devin to tell us what he knew about Michigan's new medical marijuana law. We asked him to tell us more about his experiences with marijuana, when and why and how he'd used it, how he'd acquired it, and the effect it had on him. We asked how long the effects lasted and what degree of pain relief he experienced.

Devin confessed that during a particularly hard time last summer, before we went to California, he'd started to research medical marijuana. When an opportunity to acquire cannabis had come his way, he'd given it a try. The relief had lasted about four hours and brought his pain down to about a 3 on the pain scale.

We asked him why he hadn't told us at the time, especially when his pain was getting so bad. His response was understandable: he said he didn't have the nerve to say anything. He was sure we wouldn't be supportive, given that we're opposed to the use of marijuana recreationally. He'd overheard conversations with his older brother, so he couldn't imagine our agreeing to let him use it.

The difference now was that he felt desperate. The pain was simply too much to bear. All he wanted was to leave the hospital and go home and find a way to smoke just so he could have a few hours of relief.

We talked well into the evening. We discussed the known negative side effects of marijuana as well as the unknown potential ones. Of course, in the research Devin had done, primarily on The Hemp and Cannabis (THC) Foundation sites that monopolize the search engines, he'd read that cannabis has very few side effects. He understood the side effects of smoking in general, but he was certain that cannabis either eaten or used with a vaporizer was the safest drug available for his condition. He'd found over a dozen sites supporting this notion.

Sander and I took respective deep breaths and discussed how in order to be well informed, you have to look at both sides of an argument. We told Devin we would provide him with research to the contrary so that he'd have accurate information about what he wanted to put into his body. Like any other medicine, the consumer has to understand all the risks involved, and we didn't want to go into this in an ignorant way.

Finally, late into the night, we told our son we would look into having him licensed to use medical marijuana for pain control, but that we would view cannabis just like any other medication. For starters, that meant telling Dr. Bruining and keeping her involved in the whole process.

Still tearful from his pain, Devin agreed and thanked us. He was a bit shocked at our response and confessed that he'd expected the worst.

After he was given strong medication to help him sleep, Sander and I walked out of his room like two zombies. We hugged each other in the hall for I don't know how long and then silently left the hospital for the night.

My emotions had been pulled in so many directions that day, I actually felt numb all over. All I can say, then and now, is thank god for Sander. Thank god we have one another to lean on. Thank god our marriage is so strong. The stress of this day alone, forget the whole year and a half that led up to it, would be enough to tear apart the most stable of marriages, but Sander and I have only grown closer. We haven't always agreed on how to proceed or what to try next, but through it all, we've always been able to talk to each other, listen to each other, and work together to find the best solution for Devin. We are always united in our love for one another and our love for our son. That wasn't going to change, even with medical marijuana entering the picture.

*   *   *

The next morning, after Sander went to work and Ethan and Taylor left for school, I returned to the hospital to confront whatever lay ahead. Mostly, I hoped Devin's pain had settled from the procedures of the day before. I just couldn't stand to see him endure another day at this heightened level of pain. I didn't want him to lose hope, and this was becoming the perfect scenario for him to do so. I braced myself for the worst and entered the room.

Devin had just awakened. He had slept through the night, thanks to his sleeping medications, but within seconds he was peppering me with requests to go home.

"I can't stand it here any longer; I have to go home today," turned into, "No matter what Dr. Bruining says, I'm going home today!"

His pain was hovering at a 9, and I told him Dr. Bruining just wanted him to stay until it settled, hopefully back to the 5 the ketamine had brought it to the day before. I spoke as soothingly as possible, but he was relentless. The only way I could get him to move to a new subject, even temporarily, was by reassuring him there was a possibility he could go home today.

Dr. Bruining was unable to see Devin until that afternoon, but I ran into her in the hallway. Opportunely, she wanted to sit down and talk alone without Devin present. This was good, because I needed to prepare her for Devin's downward spiraling mood, his urgent desire to leave the hospital, and his request to start using medical marijuana.

The thought of discussing this made me very nervous. I had no idea how she would respond. I feared she would be totally uncomfortable with the idea. Worse, I feared it would change her opinion about Devin and us. I had no idea how she felt about the legalization of medical marijuana in general and I didn't want to jeopardize our relationship with her. She had spent so many hours helping us; I couldn't bear the thought of her thinking we had given up and were resorting to unethical measures.

To my relief, her reaction was much like Sander's and mine the night before. She took a deep breath and, cool as a cucumber, told me she fully understood and would research the use of cannabis for pain and have a discussion about it with Devin. As the mother of a teenager herself, she immediately made me feel as if she understood our dilemma and that her heart went out to us.

After a long discussion, she knew we were not giving up on a cure for Devin and that we hoped cannabis would only be needed on an occasional basis while we continued to try other treatments and medicines.

Devin's cousins and my sister had just arrived from Chicago to see Devin. That afternoon, right before they appeared at the hospital, a group of Devin's friends showed up. This lively bunch of kids came en masse to support and distract Devin almost every day he was in the ICU, both this time and last, and some of these visits caused a stir with the ICU unit clerks because of all the fun going on behind the curtain in room 2012. In spite of this, most of the nurses were willing to let Devin's friends in to see him, even when it was against their rules, and this time was no exception.

His friends arrived around 3:15 p.m., just as Devin was starting to get upset again about leaving and repeatedly asking where Dr. Bruining was. Carefully, one of his closest friends hopped right in bed with him while the others surrounded him and began their 15-year-old antics and jokes. You could tell Devin was happy they came. I even caught a smile or two, but he was still so uncomfortable that he had a hard time enjoying their visit.

Moments later, my sister and Devin's cousins arrived, and shortly after that Dr. Bruining stopped by. Unfortunately, this meant the party had to end so she could evaluate Devin privately and discuss next steps.

She looked Devin over, talked to him about his pain level, and broke the news that she wanted him to stay at least one more night. She told him she was completely uncomfortable letting him go home in this degree of pain and in this state of mind. Somehow, amazingly, she convinced Devin to stay put one more night. He didn't even put up a fight. I guess he knew it wasn't worth the argument; she would just convince him otherwise.

We then broached the subject of what to do now. We talked about trying Trileptal, an anti-seizure drug commonly used for pain that is known to have fewer cognitive and visual side effects than Lyrica. We talked about adding another medication for sleep that also provided pain relief for many people. We discussed other medication options that could be tried if these didn't work.

To my surprise, Dr. Bruining also suggested we look further into the ketamine coma. Until now, we had pushed this dangerous, controversial procedure way back on our list of options. Frankly, we had pushed it into the "No way" section of the list.

As hard as it is to imagine, as Dr. Bruining spoke, my yearning to help Devin was so great that I began to wonder if this might be the answer after all. Just the thought of this procedure caused my heart to pound, but even the doctor we'd consulted days before had said that if his own son had been through all Devin had, he would take him to Germany for the coma.

Devin shook his head and told us flatly he'd had it with hospitals and treatments. He wasn't interested in the ketamine coma, so for the moment at least, there was no need to cross that bridge.

Acting as if I hadn't spoken with her about it, I brought up Devin's interest in medical marijuana and told Dr. Bruining we wanted her input and involvement.

She had a long talk with Devin right then and there about the potential negative cognitive side effects and possible addiction consequences of using cannabis.

Devin, of course, vehemently defended cannabis as "one of the safest drugs available" and told her he'd done plenty of research to support this.

I must say, I was impressed with how Dr. Bruining handled this rather delicate situation. She explained that the THC Foundation had overpowered the internet with their papers on the safe use of cannabis for medical reasons. She noted that it is actually quite difficult to find an article about marijuana on the internet that isn't published by the THC Foundation, but if Devin were to look harder, he would find articles by the American Medical Association and other health care organizations that discuss the possible negative consequences of using cannabis for this purpose on a regular long-term basis.

She also told Devin she knew cannabis provided tremendous pain relief for some people and that she was willing to continue the discussion and do her own research on the subject. She told him he needed to be safe and to be monitored by his parents and a physician when using any drug. Cannabis, if he were to use it, would be no exception.

The following morning, Devin rated his pain an 8. It was finally lower than the 9 he'd come into the ICU with, and I could finally breathe again. After one more visit from Dr. Bruining, he was free to unhook the ketamine and go home in the hopes that his pain would continue to settle and the new meds would kick in.

* * *

When we got home that afternoon, to no one's surprise, Devin was extremely weak. He showered and then slept for 18 straight hours. The next day, when he aroused from the dead, he told us his pain had dropped to a 7. It never returned to the 5 he had experienced just days earlier, but this was still good news. At 7, he could function. He could go to school, do his homework, and hang out with his friends.

At dinner that night, which I attempted to make a bit special to celebrate Devin's homecoming, he announced he wanted to go to school the next day. He thought he could handle it now that his pain was better. He was tired of being away from his friends and he had a lot of schoolwork to catch up on.

I didn't think this was a good idea. He was weak and tired from being bedridden for so long, but he wanted to go so badly and it was such a pleasure to see that Sander and I relented with a smile.

The next morning, Devin only made it through first hour before calling me to come pick him up. The extra walking was just too much, and he couldn't tolerate the pain.

Right then, I decided this couldn't continue. If we didn't keep him home for the rest of the second trimester, he was going to fail. He had missed 10 days while bedridden from the return of his pain following the first ketamine infusion, and seven more days while in the ICU for this last ketamine nightmare. On none of these days was he able to keep up with any schoolwork, so he was already extremely far behind.

If he kept attempting to go to school and coming home in pain, he wouldn't get anything out of these days, either. He would be useless during school and for the remainder of the day at home, learning nothing and making no headway. If he had any hope of getting caught up and passing the trimester, he would have to stay home until this trimester was over.

Devin understood. He agreed that the additional walking right now was too much. Our hope was that as we tried to get him caught up in school, we could also slowly get his strength back by re-introducing his exercise program and gradually increasing his walking. Our goal was to have him return to school in three weeks, for the start of the new trimester, and this plan worked well.

Safely ensconced at home, he was able to begin the long process of completing all his missed work from the past few weeks. His teachers understood and were helpful as I shuttled his work back and forth each day. We also got him a math tutor since he had to be taught new concepts in his advanced algebra class in order to proceed.

Thankfully, he didn't appear to have any cognitive side effects from the new medications Dr. Bruining had put him on and was as quick and sharp as usual. In time, he was able to resume his exercises and piano playing. We finally had a bit more control over this horribly uncontrollable situation, and I did my best to ignore the looming issue of medical marijuana.

Alas, Devin's terrible pain meant I wasn't able to maintain this state of ignorant bliss for long.

Chapter 9

Medical Marijuana 101

February 21, 2009

Well, it's finally here. I've avoided it as long as I could. It's time to dive into this medical marijuana issue headfirst with Devin today. There's a lot he wants to talk to me about, a lot of details he wants to share to make this a reality. It seems so surreal. I mean, he's barely 15 years old.

I know...It makes him comfortable. I know...It takes his pain away. This is all that should matter. I mean, it takes his pain away! This is really good! Then why does it bother me so much? Probably, because I know there has to be a cure out there. This will just cover up the pain! It's okay for now, but there has to be another way!

How does a mother summon up the necessary mental fortitude to face the practicalities and legalities of her 15-year-old son using medical marijuana?

Not surprisingly, Devin's research came in handy. He read everything he could get his hands on. He also contacted the head of the Michigan THC Foundation to figure out the best way to become licensed as a minor. He even joined chat rooms and was soon well connected. No one can say my son is not resourceful!

He researched issues regarding quality and value. He learned about caregivers, the licensed individuals allowed to grow and distribute marijuana to a set group of people, and about compassion groups, the support groups that exist in all communities for the purpose of networking and providing resources and up-to-date information on the legal use of cannabis. He learned, and so did we, that vaporizers were one of the safest ways for him to use cannabis.

I confess I breathed a sigh of relief when I learned there would be no smoking involved. This made it a less questionable activity, right?

Now that Devin had opened up this can of worms and felt we could have open dialogue, he wanted to share all this information with his dad and me, but mostly with me…often.

First on Devin's agenda was making sure we attended the Michigan THC Foundation's organized meeting coming up in March. Here, we would learn all the rules and regulations pertaining to medical marijuana, receive the necessary paperwork, and meet a licensed physician who would evaluate Devin and provide us with one of the two needed physician certification letters authorizing him to use medical marijuana as a minor for his chronic pain condition.

This physician came to these meetings once a month expressly for this purpose, and we needed an appointment. The law was to be instated in Michigan a few weeks after this March meeting, and a swarm of people, Devin included, wanted to be ready.

Even though any physician could evaluate Devin and provide a letter for this purpose, this meeting seemed like a good way to gain a better understanding of the process of becoming licensed to use medical marijuana. My hopes were high this doctor would have plenty of experience with the use of cannabis for this purpose and would counsel us on this issue after his evaluation, especially since Devin was a teenager.

I made the appointment, and a much relieved Devin turned his attention to another pressing issue, the purchase of a vaporizer. He told me where they could be bought locally and informed me he couldn't buy one alone because he was underage.

"Thank goodness for that," I thought. "At least they aren't readily available on the street to just anyone."

Almost immediately, I realized how silly that was. As both my sons had told me and as Devin had proven, marijuana could be scored by any teen of any age right in the comfort of their school parking lot.

*   *   *

One fine spring afternoon prior to our appointment downstate, Devin and I drove to town to view these vaporizers he'd been talking about. He took me to a small arcade of stores and we made our way upstairs to a dark and dank teen hangout. As we walked along the hallway, I couldn't help but notice the chipping paint and the 1970s carpet that looked as if it hadn't been washed since it was installed.

In addition to a few boarded up shops, we walked past a tattoo parlor, a run-down record store, a costume and magic shop, and finally the "marijuana store," as I like to call it.

As we walked in, a number of scraggly teenagers looked up guiltily. Not one of them could have been over the age of 21. In fact, the majority of those present looked to be between the ages of 14 and 18. Each kid looked at me in alarm as if they'd been caught with their hand in the cookie jar.

The store was divided into two sections. One side sold bean bag chairs, posters, and cool rock t-shirts. I guess this was the decoy for the other side of the store, which you had to be over 18 to enter. Mind you, this was a small store with a clear visual pathway from one side to the other.

This prohibited region was filled with gorgeous hand-blown glass bowls with four or five big tubes coming out of each. At first I thought they were pieces of art, very artsy vases you could give your mother-in-law on a special occasion, but fortunately I realized they were hookahs and bongs before I made a fool of myself and offered to purchase one to put flowers in.

Obviously, I'm somewhat naïve about these things. Just goes to show you, never say never when it comes to helping your child.

Devin led me to a showcase of vaporizers and summoned a nice young man – surely he was over 21? – to give us his opinion about these various machines.

I told him we needed it for medical purposes and were looking for the best one to meet this need.

As the underage kids began to quietly lurk around the forbidden area, clearly eavesdropping on our discussion, the youthful clerk very comfortably began telling us about his experience with each type of vaporizer when he gets high.

Between listening to him relay his experiences, gazing at my rapt son, and uncomfortably aware of the teenagers lingering nearby, I felt like I'd gotten stuck in a bad dream I couldn't wake up from. Was this what they called black humor? Without warning, I had a strange urge to laugh, but I contained it as best I could. I knew if my laughter broke loose, it would border on hysterical.

Devin, of course, was quite chatty on the way home. He'd been researching and knew just the vaporizer he wanted, but he agreed to wait to purchase one until after our appointment with the Michigan THC Foundation in case they had any input on which vaporizer was best.

I mentioned the possibility that they might even suggest another route for taking the cannabis that was safer and more effective for pain.

Devin agreed, and now we could put this to rest for a little while.

* * *

Unfortunately, the day came all too quickly to make the four-hour trip downstate for our appointment with the THC Foundation doctor. Although my in-laws and Sander's sister's family both lived a mere mile from where we were going, I thought it best to travel incognito. I just didn't know how I would explain what we were doing to Devin's 80-year-old grandparents or to his uncle, the rabbi.

After a nice evening hiding out at the Westin in Southfield, Devin and I awoke the next day and hurried to our early morning appointment.

To my surprise, the office was located in one of the fancy office buildings conveniently attached to our hotel. It was a lush enormous space on the twentieth floor with beautiful furnishings and huge windows overlooking the city and park.

I don't know why, but I hadn't expected this sort of ambiance. I hadn't expected the meeting to be held in the back of a multi-colored van either, but the obvious opulence struck me as humorous.

The receptionist told us to proceed to the conference room behind her. When we peeked in, I was confused – the room was filled with people who looked like they were already in the process of meeting.

At my inquiry, the receptionist explained that throughout the day, this spontaneous informative meeting would be taking place to answer questions and explain the logistics involved with becoming licensed. During this ongoing question and answer session, we would be called when the doctor was ready to see us.

Devin and I hesitatingly entered the room. The faintest aroma of marijuana reached our noses as we gazed at the mixed group of people. Some looked like hippies straight out of the 1960s and some were businessmen and women in three-piece suits. We were the only mother/son team. Not surprisingly, we saw no other minors. A video on marijuana played in the back of the room, but no one was watching it. Instead, everyone was listening to the president of the Michigan THC Foundation.

We walked in as he was discussing the legal issues pertaining to medical marijuana. We listened while he talked about who is protected and who is not and how to become and/or use a caregiver. Caregivers, we were reminded, are licensed individuals who are allowed to grow and distribute marijuana to a set group of people. If you don't grow your own, you're supposed to get the cannabis through a caregiver.

I made a mental note. We were definitely going to need a caregiver.

When I raised my hand and asked how to go about finding a caregiver, the president became noticeably uncomfortable and said that in the state of Michigan, it's illegal to discuss purchasing cannabis. This subject, he informed us, had to be discussed behind closed doors. These doors, he gestured pointedly, were wide open.

I was puzzled. If using medical marijuana was legal, why couldn't we talk about it? Further, how did we go about finding someone to talk to "behind closed doors"?

Still obviously uncomfortable, the president told me compassion groups exist in every community, and although you aren't allowed to discuss procuring marijuana within the compassion club meeting itself, you can network with other patients who come to the meeting. Nodding meaningfully, he added, "What you do behind closed doors after the meeting is no one's business."

I was immediately struck by this contradiction. On the one hand, it was legal to use marijuana as a drug for medical purposes. On the other hand, it was illegal to sell or discuss purchasing this medicine?

Quickly, I became agitated, but I still had a few questions to ask that pertained specifically to minors. I raised my hand again and explained Devin's situation.

To my surprise, the president told us that Devin would most likely have the privilege of being the only minor licensed in the state of Michigan.

This bit of information did absolutely nothing to settle my stomach, nor did hearing numerous individuals around us admit they had no medical complaints whatsoever but were simply here to be licensed to use marijuana while they had the chance.

As this was sinking in, Devin and I were called to the hall to wait for the physician. Five other people were ahead of us, but the line was moving quickly in assembly line fashion, with people walking steadily in and out of the rooms.

When it was our turn, we talked briefly to a nurse and were ushered in to meet the doctor, a clean-cut, nicely dressed gentleman in his early 60s or so. I didn't see an examining table, so I guessed he would take us to an examining room after a brief discussion once he learned more about Devin.

I seated myself and handed him the papers the nurse had given us.

We didn't exchange a single syllable and he didn't glance at Devin, much less evaluate him. Nonetheless, he picked up a pen and signed the form certifying my son as a suitable candidate to use medical marijuana.

Then he glanced at Devin and commented that he hadn't reviewed his history, even though I'd faxed it to the foundation three weeks earlier.

"So what's wrong with you?" he asked, and Devin told him he had chronic pain in his right leg from CRPS.

I asked the doctor if he knew what CRPS was and he unconvincingly said, "Yes," adding, "I'll keep some of this paperwork, and in mid-March you'll receive my official certification letter and the necessary paperwork for you to submit to the state for legal licensing."

I asked him if that was it, and he said, "Yes" and told us we could go.

I was dazed. With each passing moment, this felt more and more like a scene straight out of the *Twilight Zone* in which the main character knows something is wrong but everyone around him seems to think it's perfectly normal.

Absolutely anyone could have made an appointment with this doctor and received a physician certification letter from him, no questions asked. As a minor, Devin was required to have two physician certification letters, but this doctor was the only physician an adult needed, and hundreds of adults met with him that day alone!

It occurred to me right then and there that the legalization of medical marijuana was potentially just a scam, a great cover for the legalization of marijuana in general. Conveniently, marijuana has medicinal uses, so no doubt the grass roots effort to legalize it took full advantage of the situation. What else could explain the Michigan THC Foundation holding a mass certification weekend with this token physician?

I was disturbed for other reasons, too. Coming from a family of physicians and being a health care professional myself, I was distinctly bothered by the ethical issues of what this doctor had done. He must have made a fortune that day alone – we paid $200.00 for the privilege of having him sign his name to Devin's certification letter – and to my knowledge he didn't perform one single legitimate evaluation or explain in detail the possible side effects that come from regular usage of marijuana for medical purposes as required by the new Michigan law.

These requirements are actually written on the form the doctor signed in front of our faces. Such blatant malpractice and misuse of credentials so upset me, I vowed to contact the American Medical Society to report this physician's malpractice.

Feeling as though I were compromising my own integrity, I left the building with a terrible feeling in my stomach and the documentation that would license my son, the sole minor in the state of Michigan, to use medical marijuana.

* * *

We had a long drive back up north. After composing myself, I began a heartfelt conversation with Devin. The many issues surrounding the use of marijuana for medicinal purposes whirled through my head, but it was hard to get his adolescent mind to see why I had any concerns.

Besides his age and the undesirable social consequences that could accompany such use, I expressed how easy it could be to become dependant on this drug since it has such an immediate and potent effect on pain. I explained that even without the concern of a physical addiction, a psychological addiction was very likely since his body would crave the good feeling of pain relief again and again.

I tried to explain that this would be okay if we were at the complete end of our rope with absolutely no more ideas for treatment. If this was the case and we needed to throw in the towel, the most important thing would be functioning with less pain.

We were not at that point, I emphasized. He was young, and we probably still had more tricks in our bag, more doctors we could see, and hopefully many more interventions available.

I told Devin I was worried that if we went full speed ahead with this palliative solution, it could have a negative impact on how he viewed his pain. I worried that he would begin to see his pain as a permanent part of who he was. It could define him and take over his life. Worst of all, I was afraid he might begin to see marijuana as a necessity for the long haul and over time would lose interest in searching for a real cure.

I asked Devin to agree to start slowly and limit his use of medical marijuana to emergencies, such as when he was bumped in the leg or for an occasional break from the constant suffering. If he started off using it more generously, I told him, it would be hard to taper back.

Devin tried to understand, but he kept asking, "Why can't I just use it to make me feel better all the time? Why did we go through all this if I can't use it often to take away the pain?"

Our discussion became a bit heated, but eventually he understood that as his mother, not to mention his legal caregiver, my responsibility was to look out for his best interests. For now, this was in his best interests, and this was how we would proceed.

We also discussed logistics on our long car ride home. How would we purchase the cannabis? Who would we get it from? The foundation had explained that since Devin was a minor, a parent had to be the caregiver, i.e., provider, of the marijuana. This meant I would be licensed to grow it in our home, but I had absolutely no intention of doing so. That would completely cross the line as far as

I was concerned. After all, I had other children to consider besides Devin.

I kept thinking, "For the love of god, I drive a minivan!"

From a practical standpoint, I just couldn't see myself growing marijuana, even for medicinal purposes. Our oldest son was going through big-time teenage things and our 11-year-old daughter was right on the cusp of adolescence.

The problem was, as Devin's caregiver, I wasn't legally allowed to purchase marijuana from another caregiver. If I refused to grow it in our home, my only legal solution was to have Devin purchase it from a drug dealer at school or on the street. Oddly enough, this was somehow more legal than me purchasing it on his behalf from another caregiver!

The law is written so that, as a card-carrying patient legally licensed to use marijuana for pain control, Devin was protected. Even if he were caught in the process of purchasing marijuana from a drug dealer, the police could only arrest the dealer. Devin's card meant he was free to walk.

As his caregiver, I was not likewise protected. I could grow medical marijuana for him, but I couldn't legally buy it.

Devin and I discussed this dilemma and how we would need to talk to a lawyer who was educated in Michigan's new medical marijuana law. We also decided I would attend a compassion group meeting in our area and get a feel for the other caregivers.

In other words, legal or not, at least for the time being, I had to meet some people I could possibly "score" from.

As Devin and I retreated to our own thoughts and continued our four-hour drive back up north, I saw that my knuckles were white. The beautiful spring evening outside my window was at complete odds with the plans being concocted inside my car.

Chapter 10

A Stranger Moves In

March 16, 2009

I'm sitting at my kitchen table staring at a glass pickle jar full of "really good shit," a.k.a. one ounce of high quality cannabis buds, which I recently procured from a very nice gentleman while parked in a dark alley in the back seat of my Sienna minivan. I swear...I couldn't make this up if I tried!

It cost $200.00 and I was told this was a good price. It will probably last Devin two weeks. After that, I'll have to call the same contact and then exchange goods with my accomplice all over again.

What is so ridiculous, besides the obvious, is that I'm legally certified as Devin's caregiver, Devin is legally certified to use medical marijuana as a minor, and even my friendly accomplice is legally certified to distribute medical marijuana, yet somehow this is still an illegal activity. I feel like a common criminal with all this sneaking around. Something is very wrong here!

Anyway, I'm keeping the pickle/marijuana jar locked tightly in our file cabinet in the mud room. Unfortunately, even when it's not in use, I can smell the weed right through the jar. Somehow my home has a very different feel to it these days.

Shortly after our appointment with the marijuana doctor downstate, the third trimester of Devin's freshman year of high school began. He was strong enough now to handle the walking and was even extremely tired of spending day in and day out with his mother, but we quickly realized his new schedule was a bit ambitious.

As a result, we tweaked it so he could complete his classes by 12:45 each day without having to walk all around the huge building numerous times. He still attended his core classes and ate lunch with his friends, but a half day schedule meant he didn't overtax his leg. It further reduced his credits, but it kept him functional. He could walk, do his homework, and play lots of piano, which meant things were okay again, at least for the time being.

In dire need of a vacation and some family fun, we decided to schedule a trip to the Dominican Republic over spring break early in April. Devin's pain was holding steady at 6 ½ and he could handle it. Like the rest of us, he needed a change of scenery. We even let him bring one of his friends along, since his brother was living it up in Jamaica on his senior trip.

We stayed at a beautiful all-inclusive resort that gave Devin and his friend Eric the freedom to go at their own pace. This very large facility hosted tourists from all over the world, and it was a novel experience to be one of the only families from the United States. We met individuals from Russia, France, Italy, Spain, and Canada and decided it was a little bit like living in the town of Babel, with everyone speaking a different language.

Besides the palm trees, beautiful beaches, and great food, Devin and Eric thoroughly enjoyed the European flare, which included a slew of topless sunbathers. This exciting development had the benefit of encouraging Devin to get his exercise walking up and down the beach with Eric a couple of times each day.

Besides one rough night when Devin came down with food poisoning, our trip was a huge success until the second to last day, when Taylor accidentally hit Devin's right leg on a snorkeling boat while attempting to maneuver herself and her snorkeling gear into the water.

That was it. Devin was down and out. He lay flat on the bottom of the boat for the next hour, missing his chance to snorkel with sharks and stingrays, and then spent the rest of the day and night in his room, unable to function.

Taylor felt horrible. We all felt horrible. A simple bump on his right leg and the pain overpowered him. He recovered somewhat by the next evening, and we traveled home the following day.

*   *   *

A few days after school resumed, Devin was hit again, this time much harder, when an exuberant classmate yelled, "Yo Devin," and casually smacked him on the back of his right leg before running off to catch up with a group of friends.

I was called to pick him up, and this time I knew Devin would have a harder time recovering.

Sure enough, he missed the next day of school, and by the end of the day he was convinced his pain was worsening. With great trepidation, he told me he feared the meager benefits of the second ketamine infusion were beginning to fade.

I countered that I thought his increased pain was due to the back-to-back hits. I told him I thought he would be back on track in a day or so, but I was wrong. The next week, his pain was so bad he couldn't attend school at all, so I contacted his teachers and made arrangements to pick up his work.

At the end of the second week, Devin was still home, his pain hovering at an 8 ½. By now, he was an expert at rating his pain. He'd been asked to do so literally hundreds of times, allowing the rating scale to become extremely individualized based on his unique set-point. Sander and I trusted his accuracy and often referred to it as "Devin's Personal Pain Scale."

Though he struggled to concentrate, completing his school work was impossible, and we were forced to conclude that the slight relief he'd felt from the second ketamine infusion was indeed wearing off. What's more, the new pain medicines clearly weren't working.

We were back to where we'd been six weeks before – Devin was riddled with raw pain with no effective medicine on board. At least then, we knew he was going to be admitted to the hospital within a few days for his second round of ketamine.

Very quickly, his pain became so bad that he wanted to stay in the house and, for the first time, preferably in bed. With a sinking feeling of inevitability, we told the school we needed to change his status to homebound for the remainder of the third trimester.

We continued to push him to get out of bed, get his schoolwork done, go to his piano lesson, or even just play the piano at home, but he was in such acute, relentless pain that he often flat-out refused, and nothing we gave him provided any relief, with one exception: medical marijuana.

He could have started a plethora of new pain medications, but they all came with their own side effects, some of them truly horrific. We could have put him back on Lyrica, which kept his pain down in the 6 ½ to 7 range, but this would have sacrificed his brain and his eyesight. We could have planned for him to receive the ketamine coma in Mexico, or the new experimental three-day "close to coma" ketamine procedure being researched in Florida, but we were all leery of those options. Instead, with his pain increasingly acute, we concluded that medical marijuana was our current best option for providing him with the immediate pain relief he needed *now*.

Nonetheless, we struggled with how often to let him vaporize. Until now, his marijuana use had been limited to injuries and occasional breaks from the pain. After much discussion, Sander and I decided to let him use cannabis every other day during this difficult time.

Days he wasn't allowed to vaporize, we still insisted on certain things. He had to come to meals, not eat in bed. He had to go to scheduled appointments. He had to complete his school work. We also required him to do some walking and other exercises. We told him over and over that we would never give up on him and we would never stop looking for a cure, and he couldn't give up, either. Some of these discussions were heated. Sometimes we all cried. Sometimes we felt like we had a new, mutual understanding, only to find it had dissolved by morning.

It is so hard to think clearly when your child is in this kind of pain. Naturally, all I wanted to do was hug him, tell him everything would be all right, and bring him chicken soup in bed. It was exceedingly difficult to tell my suffering child that, in spite of his pain, he must continue with his responsibilities, but that is what we did.

These were dark days, and it was hard to know the right thing to do. Without the small amount of cannabis we let him use each week, Devin would have had absolutely no break from the worsening pain. When we did allow him to vaporize, he could do almost anything and indeed became extremely productive. For four short hours, he would catch up with his homework, play the piano, organize his room, download music onto his MP3 player, or go to an activity with the family or a friend. At these moments, all I could think was, "Thank goodness for medical marijuana."

Seeing him pain free, happy, and active literally brought tears to my eyes. He made the transition back to his happy, meaningful life so easily. He just wanted to be like any other teenage kid, hanging out with his friends and doing what teens do. It broke my heart each time I watched the pain return after this brief reprieve, but we stayed tough and continued to limit his use of marijuana in order to prevent him from becoming dependent on it.

Conversely, when we didn't allow him to vaporize, his pain was unbearable, and I was left with the helpless feeing that I could do nothing to help my child. At these times, I was tormented with guilt. How could I ask so much of him when he was suffering to this degree? How could I not allow him to use the one medicine that would relieve his pain, all of the time?

Sander and I had many sleepless nights during these months when cannabis became a fact of life in our home. As unsavory as it was to allow Devin to regularly use this substance, acquiring it made the whole experience that much more unsettling.

* * *

When none of the lawyers I contacted were able to explain the gap in the law regarding how to legally obtain cannabis, I cornered the compassion group leader at a monthly meeting one sunny spring afternoon and told him about our frustrating and ridiculous circumstances.

He said he'd heard about us; he couldn't believe the only minor in the state of Michigan licensed to use medical marijuana lived in his very own city!

For a ridiculous moment, I felt like Devin and I were celebrities. Then I asked for this gentleman's help. From whom could I purchase marijuana safely and legally? I told him I couldn't have Devin get it from his connections at school, and I wouldn't consider growing it myself. There had to be a loophole, a way for us to safely and legally buy the cannabis.

He understood our dilemma, but he knew of no legal avenue we could pursue. He was also a bit concerned about getting involved. In a very nice way, he told me he had a teenager Devin's age and that the thought of young teens using medical marijuana made him uneasy.

I told him I understood, but at this point I didn't need his opinion or judgment about what choice we had made for Devin; I just needed his help.

He told me he would look into it and get back to me.

I figured I'd never hear from him again, but he called two weeks later and said he'd found someone who was willing to act as Devin's unofficial caregiver. I asked for this person's name and number so I could contact him myself, but he told me the three of us had to meet privately to discuss the matter.

We chose a time and location one week later and met in a dark corner in the back of a bookstore in town. It was all very hush, hush, and the caregiver would only meet with me if the compassion group leader were there.

After a lengthy conversation and in spite of the caregiver's ambivalence about minors using medical marijuana, he too agreed to help us. We decided that when I needed to make a purchase, I would contact the compassion group leader and he would arrange a meeting in some dark secret place where this caregiver would climb into my car and give me the marijuana.

I was pleased to have struck a deal, but come on! It was all so sleazy! Never mind the fact that both these guys had deep reservations about giving marijuana to minors.

If Devin was protected by law and this was a legitimate medical solution endorsed by the state of Michigan, why all this sneaking around?

Nonetheless, with the help of these two kind-hearted accomplices, my brief but memorable life as a straight-laced soccer mom by day and a druggie mother scoring in dark alleys and baking marijuana brownies by night began.

*   *   *

After a month or so of using the vaporizer, Devin and I learned that eating brownies or cookies baked with carefully made marijuana butter not only provides better analgesic affects, it significantly extends the duration of pain relief, especially with nerve related pain.

Devin, in his resourceful fashion, quickly found a few marijuana butter recipes on the internet.

Resolutely facing the inevitable, I set aside an afternoon when I was certain we would have the house to ourselves for at least four hours. With Devin at the helm, we carefully followed the directions and concocted the infamous butter, but this was no easy feat! The cannabis buds first had to be finely ground and then slowly cooked with real butter in a sauce pan at an exact temperature for over an hour.

I let Devin use my coffee grinder to grind the cannabis buds, and very quickly I realized I'd made a mistake. In spite of a subsequent heavy scrubbing with hot soapy water, the small oily grains of weed stuck to the metal and the smell remained overpowering.

"Oh well," I told myself. "A new coffee grinder was in order anyway."

After being cooked, this mixture had to cool at room temperature for a number of hours and then sit in the refrigerator overnight. Once cooled in this way, I was surprised to learn that only the small green film at the top of the jelled mixture was to be used.

For a brief moment I smiled, recalling a sweet memory of my mother teaching me how to make her homemade chicken soup. This recipe also had to cool overnight in the refrigerator before the thin film of fat that congealed on top could be lifted off.

I swiftly snapped out of my revelry when I remembered this wasn't my mother's chicken soup we were making. For one thing, this concoction smelled nothing like homemade chicken soup. The buds of the cannabis plant have a potent and unforgettable aroma, one that is difficult to eliminate even with the best air freshener.

As we prepared the butter, I worried that a friend or the nice UPS man would spontaneously stop by, and I prayed the smell would disappear before Ethan and Taylor returned home from school.

Fortunately, we had no surprise visitors that day and both Ethan and Taylor went home with friends that afternoon. Our cooking complete, I hid the butter in the deep abyss of our refrigerator and did what I could to air out the house.

I awoke the next morning to birds chirping and an exceptionally beautiful day. I got the kids off to school, took a much-needed jog, did some laundry and bills, and attempted to stall as long as I could. Finally I buckled down, donned my apron, retrieved the one recipe that can't be found in the *Joy of Cooking*, and baked my first batch of marijuana brownies.

The second I took the butter from the refrigerator and unwrapped the tin foil, the pungent smell overpowered the house. I fumbled to get the other ingredients ready, hoping the cocoa and sugar would mask the smell once it was all mixed together, but it quickly became evident that nothing was going to block the fragrance of cannabis-infused butter. I even added twice the amount of cocoa and way too many chocolate chips, but it didn't work. The mixture smelled nothing like the rich chocolate smell I was used to. As I slid the pan into the oven, I gazed into the baking dish in awe. Even the typical dark brown brownie batter had a distinctly green tinge.

Alas, cooking the brownies only seemed to enhance the distinctive aroma. Once again, I began to get nervous that someone would knock at my front door. As the clock ticked away, I knew there was no possible way I could get rid of the scent by the time Taylor and Ethan returned from school. I sprayed two entire bottles of Febreze throughout the kitchen, into the living room, and around the front door, but to no avail.

Now my house reeked of brownies, Febreze, *and* marijuana.

This would be tough to explain. I took the brownies out of the oven to cool, hung up my apron, had a drink of water, and prepared myself for whatever lay ahead.

The moment Ethan came home, he gave me a high five and told me I was the coolest mom ever!

Taylor walked in and immediately asked, "What smells so funny?" Then, "Can I have a brownie?"

Devin walked into the kitchen, quietly looked over the finished product, and nodded in approval.

I told Taylor I'd made the brownies for an ill friend but I'd make another pan just for us soon. I quickly wrapped the pan up and locked it securely in an emptied file cabinet in the mud room.

I was exhausted!

*   *   *

Once, in the midst of our period of occasional trysts, this caregiver who was now providing me with the main ingredient in my new brownie recipe actually got daring and called me directly about a place to meet. When I mentioned how much I would need, he started screaming into the phone like a crazy man.

I held the receiver away from my ear, wincing. At first I didn't understand why he was upset, but then I realized he was afraid the phones might be tapped.

Once again, I asked myself what on earth I was doing. Had I really been reduced to meeting strange men in dark alleys and handing off drugs on the sly? With a vengeance, I reminded myself it was better than the alternative – having Devin procure the marijuana on his own in a parking lot somewhere.

* * *

Devin was pleased with how much better he felt when he ate a brownie versus using his vaporizer. It took his body longer to respond, since the marijuana had to be fully digested before entering his bloodstream, but once there he felt good for up to seven hours.

I must confess, I too found brownies preferable to vaporizers. When needed, I would quietly unlock the brownie vault and take a carefully measured square out for Devin to eat discretely in his bedroom.

By comparison, whenever Devin used his vaporizer, I was always on edge. He was good about using incense or heating the aromatic oils he incorporated into his snazzy new vaporizer, but no matter what he used to mask the scent, the hallway around his room always smelled of marijuana.

I would frantically spray Febreze so that his little sister, whose room was next to Devin's, wouldn't wonder what the strange smell was, but she still frequently mentioned how much she hated Devin's new incense, and could I please make him get a new type? This was a tense time for our family. Ethan was kept well informed, but it was stressful keeping Devin's marijuana use from Taylor, Taylor's friends, and the rest of our family and friends whom we were not yet prepared to enlighten. I had to constantly stay on my toes, and my worry about whether Devin would develop a dependency on this new miracle drug was draining.

Interestingly, whether he used the vaporizer or ate a brownie,

Devin never acted significantly high. His eyes became slightly bloodshot and he was happier and a little giddy, probably from a combination of the lowered pain as well as the marijuana itself, but if you didn't know he was using that day, you wouldn't have had a clue.

It was obviously a bit surreal to sit around the family dinner table knowing our 15-year-old son was high, yet it was equally heartwarming to see him happily join in the conversation, which he was never able to do when riddled with pain.

At least for now, the ends justified the means.

Chapter 11

Stumbling on the Answer

May 15, 2009

Something has to change. I refuse to believe this has become Devin's reality! Seriously, it's too sad, too ridiculous, and too painful to be true.

Today, Devin and I were eating breakfast together and laughing about Maggie and how horrible her haircut is when I accidentally kicked (more like lightly touched) his leg under the table.

Do you have any idea how hard it is not to touch or gently bump into someone you are living with or spending time with at school all day long? I have learned it is virtually impossible!

He yelled, "Mom!" and put his head down on the kitchen table, then went to his room. As usual, I felt beyond terrible. About 20 minutes later, out he came, his face gray and drawn, obviously in tremendous pain, asking for a brownie...his fourth one this week.

Will someone please wake me up? Someone out there has to know a way to make the pain of CRPS go away! There has to be someone!

One evening during this trying time, the phone rang. An old friend of Sander's, an ophthalmologist in Detroit we'd consulted about Devin's visual problems from Lyrica, was calling to tell us he'd run into an old acquaintance of his whose daughter had CRPS. She was doing great because of a program she'd recently entered at the Children's Hospital of Philadelphia, or CHOP.

When Sander told me about the phone call, I was a bit hesitant. This sounded too good to be true. By now I'd researched so many programs, I was certain I knew about every one. We'd scoured the internet almost daily month after month and had employed our impressive cadre of family physicians and physician friends to help us, to no avail. Probably this young girl had a different diagnosis and something else was going on. It felt like another wild goose chase, so I pushed the phone number aside.

Several weeks later, following a particularly difficult discussion with Devin about our decision to continue limiting his brownie intake, I decided to call this family after all. I had to find something besides marijuana that would help Devin and change the reality our lives had settled into.

By the end of my conversation with Sheryl, the mother whose daughter was in the program at CHOP, I had to admit it sounded exactly like what Devin needed.

As soon as we hung up, I logged onto the Reflex Sympathetic Dystrophy Syndrome Association's (RSDSA) web page as instructed by Sheryl. Buried among a number of different links to personal stories by different teens and children with CRPS was a video Sheryl's daughter had made titled "Alissa's Story."

I cried as I watched it. Alissa was around 15 years old and wheelchair bound at the time she entered CHOP. The emotional final scene of her video shows her running gracefully up the numerous concrete steps in downtown Philly made famous by Sylvester Stallone in *Rocky* with the theme song from the movie playing in the background.

I marveled at the change in this young lady. She and her family had been through just about everything we had, and her CRPS was worse than Devin's. If the program at CHOP developed by Dr. David Sherry had worked for her, surely it would work for Devin. The question was, how had we missed finding it?

The answer was in the terminology we collectively used. In his articles, Dr. Sherry refers to CRPS as Reflex Neurovascular Dystrophy (RND) or Amplified Musculoskeletal Pain Syndrome (AMPS). Because we'd been searching the web under Complex Regional Pain Syndrome (CRPS) and Reflex Sympathetic Dystrophy (RSD), his name never came up.

Ironically, it had also taken Alissa's family many years to find Dr. Sherry. That's why, after her daughter's great recovery, Sheryl had sent Alissa's video to the RSDS Association. Unfortunately, it had been buried as a link rather than highlighted in the youth section with a written story and picture.

*   *   *

Dismayed beyond words at the lack of coordination that delayed our discovery of Dr. Sherry, yet thrilled beyond belief to have found him at last, Sander and I devoured everything we could find on his program at CHOP. We soon learned that he looks at CRPS in a slightly different way than most physicians.

For starters, he believes that medications for pain, even herbal supplements and vitamins, hinder the retraining of the nervous system. He also frowns on medical procedures and instead urges extremely intense physical and occupational therapy while working straight through the pain, no matter how horrific.

In addition to the malfunctioning of the nerves and the constant firing of signals to the brain, he believes that patients with this syndrome have an abnormally short circuit in the spinal cord. So, while pain signals normally travel only to the brain, in patients with CRPS, these signals also travel to the neurovascular nerves that control blood flow.

This signal from the nerves causes the blood vessels to constrict, which leads to a decrease in blood flow and ultimately to a decrease in oxygen to the skin, muscles, and bone. When this happens, acid wastes like lactic acid build up, causing further pain. These new pain signals are then channeled back to the spinal column and the vicious cycle begins again, amplifying the pain even more.

Dr. Sherry believes that injury, illness, and sometimes even psychological stress can induce this abnormal reflex. He also believes the only way to break it is by encouraging normal movement and full return to function. This requires an intense amount of painful physical therapy and occupational therapy with rigorous desensitization, up to six hours a day, until this reflex normalizes.

Even after leaving his program, Dr. Sherry requires patients to take part in intense home physical therapy programs with the ultimate goal of gradually transitioning into normal daily activities with no pain.

Sander and I were struck by this approach. Without question, it was quite unique. Even if physicians treating this population don't believe that eliciting too much pain can lead to a permanent imprint on the brain (the "wind-up" phenomenon), they certainly don't routinely recommend intense and painful physical therapy and occupational therapy for six hours a day. No treatment program I'd read about up until now supported this approach, but the theory behind it resonated with me.

Without knowing it, I'd tried an extremely modified version of Dr. Sherry's program at the end of Devin's eighth grade year and throughout the summer before going to California, when he was on a three-times-a-day physical therapy schedule of swimming, biking, and exercises that forced him to work through the pain to reach new goals. At the time, I was trying to desensitize the painful area by bombarding it with normal input.

I also recall slowing way down as we read more literature, prepared to travel to California, and took to heart the warnings about the potential risk of overdoing it and potentially causing the pain to remain more permanently embedded in Devin's central nervous system.

These two conflicting approaches had caused us no end of consternation, and I'd tried to take the middle road. I was convinced that requiring Devin to do this therapy had helped prevent further loss of strength, which allowed him to remain somewhat functional and out of a wheelchair. Even so, I was nowhere close to providing him with the degree of desensitization Dr. Sherry deemed necessary.

When we found no specific doctor or program supporting the idea of pushing Devin through the pain, we'd decided to try to block it through spinal cord stimulators, medications, spinal blocks, intrathecal catheters, ketamine infusions, and the like to give his central nervous system a chance to reset and prevent the pain from becoming permanently imprinted on his brain.

Although we had some success along the way, especially after California, the greatest benefits had come from the first ketamine infusion, for the few short weeks they lasted. But after the second ketamine infusion failed, with medical marijuana moving ever more steadily into our lives, we desperately needed a fresh new angle.

We decided that Dr. Sherry's program was exactly that and we took the first appointment he had available. He had a huge waiting list, but thanks to a recent cancellation, we were squeezed in at the end of May.

Four more weeks seemed like an eternity, but the fact is, you can wait that long when you have hope, and once again we did. It was as if we knew this would be the final solution for Devin, and we itched with anticipation.

*   *   *

While we waited for our appointment with Dr. Sherry, Devin's painful daily struggle to function continued. We spent most of our time at home together, which gave me plenty of time to think about all we'd been through over the past two years as well as my physical therapy training and work with closed head injury and stroke patients.

Over the years, I'd helped many patients learn to walk again through a treatment approach called neuro-developmental treatment

(NDT). This specialized approach involves retraining the nervous system using hands-on facilitation to encourage the return of normal movement patterns.

As a student, we learned to find ways to normalize tone and posture not only during our treatment hour, but for as many hours of the day as possible so that the brain would be bombarded with this input. Plain and simple, the more patients experienced normal movement patterns; the easier it was for them to naturally begin moving this way.

I made a similar connection with individuals suffering from CRPS. Once a person succumbs to a wheelchair or crutches for an extended period of time, the brain begins to interpret this non-weight bearing status as normal. Following a painful injury, our nervous system protects us from further insult by providing an instinctive reflex to avoid using that part of the body. In most cases this is an appropriate and important reflex, which assists with healing. However, given the over-sensitized nervous system that defines CRPS, avoidance causes this reflex to intensify and becomes that person's worst enemy. It can lead to a terrible cycle of "pain and avoidance," building upon one another until the brain is convinced that not using that part of the body is the norm.

Devin avoided using his right leg by limping; his brain believed that keeping load off was the only way to control the pain. Thus, when forced to put his full weight on it, the sensation became unbearable.

I now realize how important it was that early on we didn't let him use a wheelchair. If we had, Devin most certainly would have remained in this disabled state for the long haul.

It was also becoming clear how easily medications could become a "crutch" for a patient with CRPS. When Devin stopped taking a medicine after being on it for a long period of time, his pain spiraled out of control. As with crutches or a wheelchair, his brain began to think the only way it could control the pain was with their use. This was probably what happened when his first ketamine infusion began to wear off and he was off all meds for the first time in a year and a half.

It was easy to see how the same thing could happen with medical marijuana. Unlike some medications, marijuana is in and out of your system very quickly. When it's in, it provides excellent pain control. Inevitably, it also tells the brain that pain relief is impossible without it.

In explaining this to Devin in one of our regular talks, I told him I was worried marijuana might become his "crutch." I tried to describe how, when using it, his brain could become dependent on this foreign agent as a form of pain relief and how this could hinder our ability to retrain his nervous system. Ultimately, I told him I was afraid it would prevent full, pain-free function from becoming the norm.

I reminded him of a particularly difficult two-week period when he'd begun asking to use his vaporizer more often than every other day and had told us matter-of-factly that without the marijuana in his system, his pain became much worse.

No doubt this was true. In these two weeks alone, not only was his pain unbearable when he couldn't use it, I believe he developed a psychological and most likely a physical dependency on it.

It wasn't easy, but once we came to this realization, Sander and I sat down one evening and had another tough discussion with Devin. We told him that because of these issues and given Dr. Sherry's requirement of getting off all medications before entering his program, we were going to begin weaning him from the marijuana. Initially, we would continue to allow him to have a brownie as a break from the pain three times a week, but we would gradually reduce this to zero over the next two to three months as we waited for him to enter the program.

After giving it some thought, Devin chose to have a brownie on the days he wanted to join his friends frisbee golfing. Frisbee golf, otherwise known as frolfing, is a combination of frisbee and golfing. Devin's buddies played on a wooded hilly course set up with frolf nets when not in use as a ski resort. The course is difficult, and completing one round takes hours.

Even with his special brownie on board, Devin was so weak and atrophied and his gait so slow that he could only handle about a third of the course, but he didn't care. He felt good, thanks to the brownie, and frolfing was the best exercise he'd had in a long time, not to mention the most fun.

As the weeks crept by and Devin's marijuana use slowly decreased, his pain returned, but we stuck to our guns and hoped with all our hearts that Dr. Sherry's program was the answer we'd been searching for.

* * *

By the time Devin and I flew to Philadelphia to meet with Dr. Sherry at the end of May, I was an expert at prepping Sander and the kids to be self-sufficient and I wasn't so worried about leaving them.

For their part, Sander, Ethan, and Taylor were as excited – and nervous – as Devin and I. We were all so very ready for a change. Hope had once again returned to our home, and like a breath of fresh air, it was palpable.

Ethan and Taylor had witnessed our excitement many times over the last year and a half and then just as quickly had seen it dissipate. I could feel their excitement, but I also knew they were holding back their emotions just a bit in order to avoid the letdown of watching another promising treatment vanish before their eyes.

Prior to our trip, Devin read up on Dr. Sherry's RND program and watched Alissa's video. He saw the impossible exercises she had to endure and the painful tactile desensitization the therapists performed on her six hours a day. He saw her crying and begging her therapists to please let her stop, but also her triumphant dash up the famous Rocky steps.

Truthfully, after seeing her video, I expected him to exclaim, "Are you kidding me? There's no way I'm entering a program like this!"

Instead, to my surprise, he immediately took a deep breath and said, "If they'll take me, I'll do it."

My excitement was tempered with anxiety at the thought of meeting Dr. Sherry. Given how many bad experiences we'd had with new doctors, I just couldn't bear to hear another physician say Devin didn't have CRPS because his leg wasn't red or cold during the visit.

Over and over, my thoughts returned obsessively to the same questions. Was Dr. Sherry going to be one of those doctors who wanted the parent to remain silent while he talked with the child? Would he make quick judgments about Devin and me? Would he conclude I was overbearing and burdened with marital problems that had caused deep psychological issues to develop in our son?

I was completely scarred from our bad experiences in Wisconsin and elsewhere, and I really hoped we wouldn't have a repeat with Dr. Sherry.

* * *

I was pleasantly surprised when a short older man with a long grey beard wearing black converse sneakers and a playful tie walked into the examining room. After spending over an hour talking with Devin and me and listening carefully to Devin's story, he began doing a load of magic tricks and telling riddle after riddle to Devin. Amusing, yes, but also a good way for him to assess Devin's concentration and how pain affected it.

Dr. Sherry then informed Devin that he had to assess his right leg and he wasn't going to baby it. He was going to move it and press it the same as he would his left leg. He told Devin he knew this would hurt and that it was a little bit of a preview of what to expect if he were to enter his program.

Devin was prepared for this, but that didn't make it any easier. I don't know if it was harder for Devin to endure or for me to watch as Dr. Sherry, not so gently, evaluated his leg for a full 15 minutes.

Devin's face turned grey and tears quickly began running down his cheeks, but he never screamed or asked Dr. Sherry to stop.

Immediately after his evaluation, Dr. Sherry went right back to his magic and riddles, but this time there was no reaction from Devin. He couldn't answer any riddles, even the ones Dr. Sherry had told him earlier, and he didn't smile at the magic. When the pain was this agonizing, he predictably became silent and stone-faced.

I cannot begin to describe my feelings when Dr. Sherry informed us the program was perfect for Devin. I had to physically stop myself from jumping up and hugging Dr. Sherry and lifting him off the ground. Fortunately, I had a bit of self control, because I am much taller than him and I could have done it with ease.

Dr. Sherry explained that at least 30% of kids have a reoccurrence of their CRPS after leaving the program, usually induced by an illness, a sprain, or a broken bone, but he noted that at least half of this subgroup would be able to use the desensitization skills and exercises they learned at CHOP to reverse their pain on their own. If they couldn't do it on their own, some would be readmitted for a second go-around.

Before we left, Dr. Sherry showed Devin a simple medical diagram of the normal pain pathway within the nervous system. He told Devin his pain was absolutely real, no matter what anyone had insinuated in the past, and he went on to explain what was going wrong within his spinal cord and associated nerves. He showed him the abnormal reflex and explained how intense physical and occupational therapy worked to override it.

The only bad news was that Dr. Sherry couldn't guarantee Devin would be admitted to the program this summer. The waiting list was long, and every child had a personalized plan. Some only stayed two weeks, but others stayed six, depending on how quickly they responded.

We would have to wait a minimum of several more months to begin the program that would simultaneously cause Devin tremendous pain yet give him back his life, but waiting had become a way of life for us. I felt certain the program would help Devin, and I kept reminding myself, "What are a few more months if we're finally on the right track?"

Even Devin, in brief one-syllable grunts following his painful evaluation by Dr. Sherry, conveyed how glad he was to be accepted into his program. After being manhandled a few minutes prior, I truly wasn't sure what his reaction would be, and I was elated to hear he was still on board.

*   *   *

Shortly after our return to Traverse City and greetings from an ecstatic father and siblings, school ended. Because Devin had spent most of the last trimester at home, he finished with A's and B's. In addition, because of my success with the gym credits, he managed to leave the ninth grade only one half credit short.

His biggest challenge, now that it was summer, was to finish slowly getting off all his medications, a requirement prior to starting Dr. Sherry's program. This included Deseryl, which he was taking to help him sleep as well as the limited marijuana he was still using.

We didn't tell Dr. Sherry about the cannabis. Sander, Devin, and I decided that since he would be finished with it by the time the program began, there was no need to burden Dr. Sherry with this information. Call us cowards, but we had no way of knowing how he might respond, and we didn't want to jeopardize our relationship with him.

Devin agreed to a plan of cutting back every two weeks until he was off the marijuana completely, even if he was injured and in excruciating pain. He understood what he had to do and why, and in spite of a few minor injuries over the next few months, he followed through until medical marijuana, mercifully, was out of our lives for good.

As June progressed, to our surprise, Devin's pain slightly decreased. By the end of the month, he was even well enough to plan a well-earned piano recital at our home with both his classical and jazz teachers as well as family and close friends. In total, over 60 people attended.

Ethan and Taylor and even some of Devin's friends helped set up the day before. We were all excited. As I quietly counted away the minutes, I crossed my fingers that Devin wouldn't stub his toe or hurt his leg in the next 24 hours.

Of course, I should have known better. The evening before his recital, while maneuvering through the maze of chairs that now filled our entire first floor, Devin stubbed his toe on the side of a chair.

I heard his scream and found him flat on the ground, writhing in agony.

As always, my heart sank and my joyful disposition deflated. I envisioned having to make a last-minute call to his piano teachers and all our friends and family telling them the recital was cancelled. Everyone we'd invited had witnessed Devin's incapacitation from minor injuries such as this and would have understood, but I just didn't want to do it.

Devin had already eaten his allotted brownies for the week, but it only took a few moments for Sander and I to agree this was an exceptional situation.

Later that evening, when the extra brownie had taken effect, Devin emerged from his bedroom, gave us each a hug, and told us that if his pain was down by morning, he still wanted to perform.

The next day came, and Devin played beautifully, probably better than he'd ever played before. He entertained us on the rebuilt 1886 ebony Steinway his grandparents had given him years before with 45 minutes of lovely classical and heartfelt jazz tunes including "Lullaby of Birdland" by George Shearing, "My Funny Valentine" by Richard Rodgers, "'Round Midnight" by Thelonious Monk, "Rachmaninoff Prelude in G Minor Op. 23, No. 5," and a beautiful Mozart Concerto duet with Dr. Coonrod, his classical teacher.

All told, he brought this warm, supportive crowd to a standing ovation. Everyone understood what an accomplishment it was for him to play so well, and he was surrounded by love.

*   *   *

Devin's pre-recital injury aside, we wondered what had caused his pain to diminish. He attributed it to his past use of medical marijuana and reminded us that when we allowed him to use it, he was much more active and exercised at a higher level, which made him stronger and more functional.

This was certainly true. With cannabis in his system, he could exercise much harder, take long walks, and hike long distances through the hilly terrain of the frisbee golf course.

Looking back, the three days each week he ate a brownie and exercised at this level of intensity were extremely therapeutic both psychologically and physically. Devin gained strength and agility, and perhaps this is why his pain began to decrease.

All that mattered now was that he was in good shape to begin Dr. Sherry's program, but when I say "in good shape," I should clarify. He was still suffering, was extremely weak, and had lost agility, speed, and muscle mass. The difference was, he was no longer incapacitated by his pain. He was once again interested in joining his friends and our family in activities, as long as he didn't have to walk too much and his leg wasn't touched.

For example, a week after his recital, Devin accompanied a group of friends to see the annual 4th of July fireworks on Grand Traverse Bay. I feared he would find the sandy beaches too difficult to navigate and that he might get bumped as he walked among the crowd, but I also knew his friends would take good care of him. Numerous times, I had seen them huddled around him to create a barrier and walking at painstakingly slow speeds to stay with their buddy.

I agreed to pick Devin and his friends up after the fireworks. As most of the crowd dispersed, I waited patiently at our designated meeting spot as hundreds of people passed by and the crowd thinned.

I knew Devin would be slow, but as time passed, I began to worry. Was the distance too much? Had he been hurt?

Moments later, I spotted a scraggly group of kids walking towards me, slower than turtles, laughing and smiling. Devin was in the middle, grimacing with each step he took, but clearly happy.

*   *   *

We waited for the call from CHOP all through the summer. It wasn't easy, but we tried not to obsess on when it might come and instead spent our time swimming, sailing, eating hot dogs at the beach, building bonfires, and enjoying Ethan's last summer home before he went off to college.

The third week of August, the phone rang and we learned that Devin would begin Dr. Sherry's program on August 31, one week before the beginning of his sophomore year of high school.

I took a deep breath, beset by the conflicting emotions of excitement, relief, and a tinge of dismay that, once again, Devin was going to miss a huge chunk of school.

I shook that thought away and concentrated on the positive. He was about to enter the program that would finally end his pain and give him back his life. We had much to be grateful for.

Chapter 12

From Tears to Triumph

August 28, 2009

It's my birthday! I'm 47 today. Truthfully, I'm a bit too stressed to fully appreciate everything Sander and the kids did for me today. Of course, they were wonderful. They made me breakfast and got me flowers and treated me special all day long like usual.

It's just that Devin and I leave for Philadelphia in two short days and I still have a lot to do! I have so many arrangements to make for Taylor, bills to pay, packing to do, and loads more things to get for Ethan before he leaves for college. I don't know if it's even humanly possibly to get all this done. I just wish we knew how long Devin and I were going to be gone. I think it would make things a bit easier. Maybe once I fill in the huge calendar with a big red marker for Sander with all the things he has to remember, I'll feel better.

I spent a big part of the day helping Ethan get organized for college. Oh my god! His room was such a disaster! I, of course, told him to go through it beforehand, but this obviously didn't happen. Digging through and deciding what should stay and what should go gave me such a headache. I don't know how, but right when I thought I was going to lose it, he somehow managed to make me laugh so hard I started crying to the point where my stomach actually ached. He has a gift, my son, and this I will miss with him away.

Well, I'm exhausted. I have to go to sleep so I can be productive tomorrow. We leave early the following day, so I've got to be on my toes in the morning.

I have a feeling my 47th is going to be a good year. I have a really good feeling that our nightmare is about to end, and I have a really good feeling about Dr. Sherry's program at CHOP. I can't wait for Devin to get started!

After equal parts planning, arranging, and anticipating, Devin and I flew back to Philadelphia on Sunday, August 30, 2009.

My emotions were decidedly mixed. Ethan was starting college at the University of Michigan on September 2, and I wouldn't be home to take him or help him move in. I prepared him the best I could, but it was hard not being there as my first son went off to college.

Taylor was starting middle school the following week, but I wasn't as worried about this transition. She was familiar with the setting, having watched her brothers go to the same school, and she was excited about soccer season, starting classes, and seeing her friends. I had worked feverishly to make sure she was prepared with school supplies, after-school plans, and the like before we left, and the thought of her brother getting better was so thrilling, she was actually happy to see us go.

Sander was fully prepared too, thanks to the huge calendar labeled "Everything You Need to Know about the Weckstein House" that detailed Taylor's carpools, after-school activities, bus route, and the various phone numbers and bills he'd need to be on top of while we were gone.

Until now, three weeks was the longest we'd been away. Needless to say, by the time we left, I felt as organized as humanly possible given that I was leaving my husband and daughter and our valiant, patient Maggie to fend for themselves for god knew how long.

* * *

Devin and I lived at the Ronald McDonald House in Philadelphia for the duration of his outpatient program at CHOP. The very first Ronald McDonald House in the world, this very old building was originally a prominent family's mansion and later was expanded to accommodate up to 45 families. Devin and I shared a decent-sized room with two double beds and a TV. To our delight, everything we needed was on hand, from desktop computers to hair dryers to laundry detergent.

Washers, dryers, and soda machines were set at a quarter, and evenings were occupied with art projects, visits from area shelter dogs, and various activities and entertainment. For a $15.00/day donation per room, basic food for breakfast and lunch was provided in the kitchen at all times, with dinners made nightly by volunteers from the community.

I was truly impressed. What piece of mind not to have to worry about finances while Devin was being treated. Our lodgings were old and a bit mildewy, and several families shared common bathrooms in the hall, but that didn't matter. The Ronald McDonald House was a safe, caring, and very special place, with no questions asked as far as how long you needed to stay.

Like us, a number of the families we met at the Ronald McDonald House had children in the hospital at CHOP. These many anxious, exhausted parents and their children – some waiting for surgeries, others sporting bald heads and clearly fighting cancer – left quite an impression on Devin and me.

As we checked in, I noticed a young girl gimping around on her right leg and holding her mom's hand. It was glaringly obvious that she, too, was here for Dr. Sherry's program.

For the first time, it hit me that Devin wasn't alone. There were others out there just like him. After two years of dealing with CRPS basically on our own, it seemed surreal to see someone else struggling with this problem.

*   *   *

Devin and I used public transportation during our stay in Philadelphia based on a recommendation by Alissa's mom, Sheryl. They happened to be in Philly for a follow-up appointment with Dr. Sherry, so they came to the Ronald McDonald House the evening we checked in to meet us and cheer Devin on.

Alissa was now 18 and extremely sweet and friendly. She'd been in the program for eight weeks initially and then for another three weeks after a second broken ankle and a redevelopment of her CRPS. She'd just been released from her local hospital after recovering from a rather mysterious illness. She and her mom had seen doctor after doctor, and they were here to ask Dr. Sherry if he thought this new problem might be a form of CRPS.

It made me a bit nervous for Devin to learn all this the evening before he started at CHOP, but he just appreciated meeting someone else with CRPS who'd had a great response in the program and his attitude stayed positive.

A quote by Lance Armstrong nicely summed up Devin's mindset on this memorable day: "Pain is temporary. It may last a minute, or an hour, or a day, or a year, but eventually it will subside and something else will take its place. If I quit, however, it lasts forever."

During an especially difficult time last year when Devin's visual and cognitive problems had been at their peak, we'd encouraged him to listen to Lance Armstrong's book on tape, *It's Not about the Bike*. This inspirational story had hit home. Devin was struck by Lance's courage and relentless determination to fight through his cancer, and he shared Lance's view on not giving in and never giving up.

* * *

The next day, Devin's first day in Dr. Sherry's program, we woke up early, slowly walked two painful blocks to the nearest bus stop, and found our way to CHOP and the third floor where Devin would begin his RND program. Promptly at 8:00 a.m., after a brief evaluation by

Deb, the nurse practitioner and Dr. Sherry's main sidekick, Devin was whisked away and I was on my own.

I made the best of the situation by getting my bearings. I learned about the bus routes, the city, places to eat and grocery shop, and good places to jog. To calm my nerves, I went for a long run along the Schuylkill River that divides University City and Center City. The hospital was on one side of the University of Pennsylvania campus and the Ronald McDonald House was on the other, and I took the first of many walks through this beautiful Ivy League campus.

Devin's first day in the program was just as I'd expected. When I picked him up at 4:00 p.m., he looked as if he'd been run over by a Mack truck after running a full marathon. With his hair soaked through with sweat, his face bright red, and his shoulders slumped, he could barely limp up the last step to the third floor and into the waiting room where I was to meet him.

Silently and very slowly, he limped his way out of the hospital and back down the three flights of stairs to the bus stop outside CHOP a block away. He had to find a way to keep going. Starting today, he wasn't allowed to use elevators in the hospital; he was to use the stairs at all times.

Once back in our room, after a quick shower and firmly planted in bed for the remainder of the evening, he told me about his day. He'd been evaluated for six hours, with a one-hour break for lunch and one hour of free time. He'd performed a difficult treadmill test that required him to walk or run for as long as possible as the speed and grade were progressively increased. He'd climbed five flights of stairs and performed dozens of different animal walks and a slew of timed activities. His ability to jump and run had been evaluated, his leg had been rubbed down with a towel and ice, and he'd been introduced to the dreaded Shaker, a machine that vibrated with great intensity on his right leg.

The therapists were nice, but they expected him to do better with each attempt. He said that even though he'd tried his hardest not to, he couldn't help groan, let out a few screams, and even cry at times.

He also told me he'd never once told them to stop, even though every possible thing he'd tried to avoid for the past two years had been inflicted upon him that day, over and over again.

Remarkably, as my exhausted son told me about his horrific day, he never became obstinate or angry. He never once mentioned not going back the next day, how he hated the therapists for what they'd done to him, or what a stupid program this was. As a matter of fact, not one single swear word came out of his mouth. He was ready, resolved, and determined to withstand whatever they threw at him. This was his last hope, and he was going to endure it.

I was amazed at his level of focus and sheer will, especially when I recalled his typical reaction at home or school after being hit in the leg. He seemed to have completely embraced the program's philosophy, agreeing to tolerate extra suffering in the weeks ahead if this could take away his pain for good.

Devin rose the next day in excruciating pain after a sleepless night. Still, he muscled through the early morning with no complaints and limped into the hospital determined and ready to go.

As an indication of how committed he was to making this program work, Devin used the stairs that day and every day thereafter everywhere we went, even outside the hospital.

To say I was proud of him is the understatement of the century.

That morning, while we waited for his therapies to begin, I met two of the other kids in the program, including the girl we'd observed the day we checked in.

Anna was eight. She had pain primarily isolated to her foot that also originated from a sprained ankle. Her limp was severe, and she'd lost most of her normal function in that leg.

Morgan was nine years old and had burning, stabbing pain in her foot, left wrist, and right fingers that had spread to her face and stomach. Her CRPS had begun from a series of bad luck including a sprained ankle, a broken wrist on one hand, and a broken finger on the other. Although she felt a lot of pain, she was completely functional. She had a slight limp, but she could run and jump and ride her bike.

Like Anna, she'd sustained her original injury and then developed CRPS recently, fewer than four months ago. Both girls were from Philadelphia, and their doctors were from CHOP. They'd recognized the early signs of CRPS and had the girls scheduled for appointments with Dr. Sherry almost immediately.

Anna and her mom were staying at the Ronald McDonald House, but Morgan and her mom took a train to CHOP each morning, which meant they had to wake up every day at 4:30 a.m. to catch the train and didn't return home until almost 7:00 o'clock each night. This soon became wearisome, with Morgan in tears each morning and Laurie frazzled and upset, so they too began staying at the Ronald McDonald House.

This was the beginning of a unique and lasting friendship between Devin and his little girlfriends and the other two moms and me. Very much like brothers and sisters, Devin consoled Anna and Morgan when they cried, and the girls waited for him as he slowly made his way up the three flights of stairs after therapy each day. They saw each other face seemingly impossible challenges, and they provided words of encouragement that got them through what only they could understand.

*   *   *

At first Devin and I took the city bus to the stop three blocks from the hospital each day, but soon Anna's mom, Rachel, graciously began driving us each morning.

After dropping Devin off, I usually went for a long run and explored different parts of the city and various historical sites including the Liberty Bell, Constitution Hall, Old Town, Penn's Landing, and Rittenhouse Square.

While I was roaming the streets of Philly and enjoying the beautiful old architecture, here's what Devin was up to:

Pool therapy 8:00-9:00 a.m.
Physical therapy 9:00-10:00 a.m.
Occupational therapy 10:00-11:00 a.m.
Physical therapy 11:00-12:00 p.m.
Lunch 12:00-1:00 p.m.
Occupational therapy 1:00-2:00 p.m.
Occupational therapy 2:00-3:00 p.m.
Physical therapy 3:00-4:00 p.m.
Occasional art or music therapy from 4:00-5:00 p.m.

At first, he could do very little. When asked to walk on the treadmill, he could only last a few seconds on a level surface at the slowest speed, around 1.5 mph. It took him 14 minutes to painstakingly go up and down five flights of stairs. He could lift his legs in and out of a bathtub six times in one minute.

In addition to brutal exercises including the stand-sit bike, elliptical, treadmill, strength training exercises and machines, aquatic therapy, Pilates, and mat work, Devin's therapists immediately began setting up grueling timed activities for him that he was asked to beat each day. These included funky animal walks down a long hall like the inch worm, the crab, the three-legged dog, and the kangaroo. If he didn't beat his previous day's times, he had to repeat them until he did, even if it took all day.

In addition to the Shaker, he also received pure desensitization a minimum of twice a day with something called a Thumper, which had two flaps that beat up and down on his leg. He also somehow managed to endure a daily ice massage of his leg two to four minutes each day before the team decided it was just too hard for him to bear and would be reintroduced at a later time.

Dr. Sherry and Deb came into the gym every morning to say hello and do a quick assessment of the kids. Dr. Sherry would dance with each of the girls and joke with the boys; he always left each of them with a random interesting fact he asked them about the following day. I presume this was his way of simultaneously evaluating their present state of pain and its effect on their cognitive abilities and having fun with the kids. They all adored him and greatly looked forward to his daily rounds.

After the first week, one of Devin's therapists began repeatedly hitting him in the right leg with a rubber bat and stepping on his right foot. I'm certain she included this since we'd relayed how incapacitated Devin became at home if he were hit in the leg.

The therapists were young, energetic, and friendly yet somehow they managed to impose this daily torture on the kids while remaining encouraging and sweet. Not surprisingly, it took them a long time to really get to know Devin. For at least the first week, they thought he was reclusive, shy, and perhaps a bit unfriendly.

I knew they were seeing my son in his stone-faced and shut-down state of mind, just trying to survive, but as the weeks went by and he became more accustomed to their expectations and the pain he endured, his true personality came out and he charmed each of them with his gentle, talkative, and friendly demeanor.

* * *

His first week, Devin left the hospital each day completely spent. He took a shower, ate a quick meal, and went straight to bed.

By the end of week one, he was making a brief appearance in the dining room for dinner with Anna and Morgan before retreating in exhaustion to our room.

By the end of the second week, our three families were eating dinner and spending time together each evening.

Not unexpectedly, sometime during that first week, Devin's pain worsened and began to spread, first into his left leg and foot, then into both arms. His autonomic nervous system was on overdrive, but we'd been warned it would get worse before it got better, so this wasn't a surprise.

The nerve fibers responsible for sending pain signals to the brain from his right leg were already highly sensitized from his CRPS, firing rapid and constant pain signals to his brain. With the further insult from the program, they became even more sensitized.

I explained to Devin that with the increase in hyperactivity of the nerves, a build-up of chemicals can occur in the space between the neurons. What can't be reabsorbed often spreads to nearby sections of the spinal cord, which can lead to over-activity of the neurons, causing pain to spread to other areas of the body. Typically, this happens in the areas closest to the original insult, which in Devin's case meant his left leg.

This explanation made sense to Devin, but it provided little comfort. He was the one who had to deal with his nervous system going haywire and his pain spiraling out of control. He was unmistakably miserable, but the more Devin's therapists inflicted on him, the more confident I became. I knew this was the only way to truly desensitize him. Being ultra careful at home and trying to prevent injuries had only made things worse. His nervous system had simply become far too used to avoiding what should have been normal sensations.

Fortunately, because we had Dr. Sherry's encouragement and expertise, we knew we were doing the right thing, and this allowed Devin to muster up the strength and resolve to endure it.

*   *   *

Each evening after dinner, Devin and I called home. I would catch up with Taylor, Devin would relay the day's hard-earned accomplishments to his dad, and then I would go into the hall and privately talk with Sander about how pleased I was with the program yet how scared I was that it might not work.

Two and a half weeks into it, Devin's pain had not only spread into his left leg and arms, it was still considerably worse than when we'd arrived. He was making slow but steady progress with strength and agility, but I was anxious for his pain to abate.

I tried to push it into the deep dark recesses of my mind, but small twinges of doubt began to surface. He'd been so resistant to so many treatments; what if this too didn't work?

It was always helpful talking with Sander on these lonely nights. He would reassure me from afar that everything would be all right, and somehow he would convince me that while this was going to take time, surely Devin would respond.

*   *   *

The weekends came as a big treat for Devin. He still had to do a 45-minute exercise program twice a day as well as the homework his teachers were kind enough to fax every few days to the Ronald McDonald House, but this was nothing compared to what he'd been going through all week.

We'd heard about the Reading Market, pronounced "Redding," a huge indoor farmers' market with small restaurants and shops. To our delight, we learned this market was the inspiration for the Reading Railroad property on the Monopoly board. Devin's therapists gave us all sorts of recommendations about which places to visit, like the Amish Bakery for pretzels and Delilah's for their famous fried chicken.

On our first visit, we ate until we were practically sick. We gorged ourselves on oatmeal cookies, ice cream from the oldest ice cream vendor in the country, and of course pretzels and fried chicken.

We also took the city bus to Old Town to see a couple of movies, and once we digested our Reading Market binges, we found great places to have dinner. On the Jewish New Year, Rosh Hashanah, which happened to fall on a weekend this particular year, we rented a car and spent the day with close friends in Baltimore.

These outings helped us forget the trauma of the week and face with a bit more grace those that lay ahead.

*   *   *

Slowly, Devin's strength and stamina increased. He began walking at slightly faster speeds on the treadmill for longer periods of time, he became faster at going up and down the five flights of stairs, and he consistently beat his animal walks and the other timed activities they threw at him.

All of this was good, but I was really excited when, at the end of week three, he told me he'd jogged a short distance for the first time. I could hardly believe my ears, and I begged him to show me. Running, much less jogging, was something he hadn't done in two years!

After much pleading on my part and a bit begrudgingly on his, he ran 20 feet or so. He looked a bit awkward and it was clearly painful, but he ran!

Most of us take running for granted, but it requires significant strength and coordination of multiple muscles in the leg and foot, which must then be properly integrated by the nervous system. In spite of our best efforts, Devin's muscles had become so atrophied that, until now, running was literally an impossible feat. What success to have the strength and balance to be able to launch off his right leg!

My excitement was matched only by my jealousy of Devin's therapists. I didn't want to take over or even be a part of his therapy; I simply wanted to watch. After all we'd been through, it was hard to take a back seat and hear about his accomplishments after the fact. I knew it wasn't a good idea to have me watch, but I often wished I had a hidden camera.

My weekly meeting with Deb each Thursday was my only lifeline to Devin's therapy. At times, she spent an entire hour talking with me about how things were going and the progress he was making. She was quite smitten with him, and she often commented that she'd rarely seen a child so determined to get better. Once he could run, she told me, his therapists had reintroduced other functions his body had all but forgotten such as hopping, jumping, sprinting, jump rope, and even a little tennis.

Predictably, Devin staggered up the steps from the gym at the end of each day covered with sweat, and his daily description of what he'd done floored me. On one particular day, during the last hour of physical therapy, he'd been asked to ride the bike for 15 minutes and get to a certain distance by that time. If he didn't make it, for every extra minute it took him to get there, he had to walk backwards on the treadmill one more minute.

The first time, it took him three extra minutes to reach the required distance, so he was required to do three minutes of backwards walking on the treadmill. This alone wouldn't have been so bad, but he had to repeat the goal on the bike until he succeeded in reaching the distance in the required time.

In between each failed attempt, after the backwards walking on the treadmill, he had to do two minutes of timed double leg and single leg jump rope as well as 10 squat jumps and three flights of stairs.

Since it took Devin three tries on the bike to get to the distance his therapist assigned him, he earned an additional 45 minutes on the bike, 30 squat jumps, six minutes of timed jump rope, nine flights of stairs, and five minutes of backwards walking on the treadmill before he was allowed to leave the gym.

Mind you, this was just one of the six intense hours of physical therapy and occupational therapy he had each day, with both his right and left leg feeling the constant burning pain of CRPS!

For anyone to willingly embrace this sort of punishment was difficult to imagine, and I was grateful Devin had the maturity to understand what was at stake. This was a harder task for Anna and Morgan, but Devin was always there to encourage them. At one point when Morgan was having an extremely hard time, crying as she left her mom at the hospital door and through most of her morning therapies, Devin offered to let both girls paint his nails that evening at the Ronald McDonald House if they would try their best not to cry as they left their moms the next morning.

Crying as they went through their therapy was another story. Even Devin shed tears when his leg was forcibly patted down or during the last 30 seconds of some dreadful workout, so not crying during therapy wasn't part of the bribe.

It took some thinking, but the girls finally agreed, and Devin showed up at therapy the next day with two giggly girls and rainbow-colored nails for all to see.

I watched the goodness in my son shine and felt so proud of the young man he had become.

*   *   *

At the end of week three, Devin began to sense that if he continued to progress, he was close to going home.

Strangely enough, this worried me. His strength and function were still far from normal. The pain in his right leg was still higher than when we'd arrived, and though the arm pain had gone away, he still had the new pain in his left leg.

He couldn't run functionally yet, in terms of participating in a real activity like tennis. He couldn't walk fast enough for long enough periods of time to keep up with his friends as they Frisbee golfed. He was much, much better, but he still had a long way to go in terms of strength, balance, and muscle re-education.

I worried all weekend, thinking about all we'd been through, how far we'd come, and all we'd sacrificed to be here. I so badly wished Devin could get every possible benefit from this program before we went home.

When Devin woke up on Sunday morning, he had some thrilling news: for the first time since we'd arrived, his pain had dropped.

To finally hear these words with no assistance from medications, implants, blocks, or ketamine was simply miraculous. Now more than ever, I wanted him to stay, to see what they could get out of him before we had to leave.

On Monday morning, I called Deb to express my concern. I told her that the more functional and the stronger Devin became before we left, the better his chances of success once he went home. In spite of his newly decreased pain and his newfound ability to jump, I told her I didn't think he'd gotten over the hump yet.

I told her I needed to feel that, once discharged, he could continue to progress at home. I knew all too well how tedious a 45-minute exercise program could be in terms of seeing steady gains. Right now, I felt that if we relied too much on him doing a home program once a day, he would begin to slide backwards.

He was going to be bombarded with school work once we got home, I explained, and he would want to play the piano. Most importantly to him, he would want to return to being the extremely social boy he'd always been.

Deb understood my concerns and reassured me that Devin's team had no current plans to discharge him at the end of the week. She said they would consider all facets before recommending discharge from the program, especially given how far he lived from Dr. Sherry and CHOP.

Our conversation made me feel better, and I left it in their hands. They'd brought more than a thousand kids through the program to date; they knew what they were doing. I just had to trust their decision when the time came.

* * *

Week four turned out to be a huge turning point for Devin. During this week, he began to run. He started out jogging on the treadmill two minutes at a time with a one-minute walk break for 10 to 15 minutes at 4.6-5.0 mph. He progressed quickly all week until he could run up and down five flights of stairs in one minute and 37 seconds.

By comparison, when he'd started the program, it had taken him 14 minutes to run five flights of stairs.

By Friday, he was doing suicides, intense sprints back and forth on a tennis court or gym, each time going a farther distance and then back again.

As he ticked off his accomplishments each night, I just shook my head. The week before, he'd only just begun to jog. Decreased pain and increased strength were a marvelous combination!

That Thursday, during our weekly meeting, Deb confirmed that they were going to keep him one more week for his fifth and final week. The team wanted to get him in the best possible shape before he went home and had carefully discussed all he'd been through before making their decision.

I was delighted. Devin was progressing so quickly; who knew what he could do if he had one more week of hardcore therapy? As a fringe benefit, this also meant we had one more weekend at the Ronald McDonald House, one more city bus ride to the Reading Market for fried chicken and ice cream, and at least six more episodes of *It's Always Sunny in Philadelphia*, a totally mindless, fairly inappropriate, and completely hysterical sitcom we'd been watching each night since we'd arrived.

*   *   *

That Sunday, I again woke up to great news: Devin's pain had once again dropped. He was now at a 4 on the pain scale and felt ready to go home. He was confident he could handle anything that came up. He was no longer worried about getting bumped at school; he knew he could handle it. Likewise, he was certain he could keep up with his friends in anything they chose to do. Knowing he had the ability to work through the pain, no matter how bad it became, was liberating.

"I might even be faster than they are now," he told me with a grin.

I had to laugh out loud at the look on his face. It was so good to have my funny, charming, occasionally devilish son back. To hear him this positive and happy was a sure sign he was going to be okay. I hadn't seen him look like this since he was 13 years old, and as I gazed into his hazel eyes, I could feel two years' worth of weight slowly lifting from my shoulders.

Devin could practically taste his freedom, but he had a hard and brutal week ahead of him. As I look back, it's absolutely crazy what he accomplished his final week at CHOP. He left Dr. Sherry's pain program able to jog 6.4 mph at a 22% incline while running for 18 minutes and 30 seconds on the treadmill in the performance test that progressively increases speed and incline of the treadmill for as long as the participant can tolerate it. For comparison's sake, his first week, he could stay on the treadmill for only 16 *seconds* slowly walking at 1.5 mph with the treadmill at a 0% incline.

During his last stair climbing test, he ran up and down the five flights in 34 seconds, skipping steps along the way. He jumped rope over a hundred times on two legs and even a few dozen times just on his right leg.

There were a thousand more accomplishments, but most importantly, he left able to endure being whacked on the right leg over and over again and come out of it smiling, ready to run around the gym and whack that person back. This ability to respond in kind, not surprisingly, was seen by the therapists as a clear sign the patient was on the mend, and they learned to watch out!

*　*　*

Our last day at CHOP was quite emotional. For the first time since our arrival, I was allowed to enter the physical therapy gym, watch Devin's last hour of therapy, meet all five of his therapists, and say goodbye to Deb and Dr. Sherry.

Devin had grown very close to each therapist and had a gift and his own special words for each of them.

In turn, his therapists told me over and over again how they rarely encountered a child as motivated as Devin. During the most difficult of times, in spite of tears and agony, he never said, "I can't." He'd worked extremely hard to climb his personal mountain, and they knew it.

Dr. Sherry gave Devin a big hug, told him how proud he was of him, and said he looked forward to hearing about Devin's progress at his one-month, six-month, and then yearly follow-up appointments.

After our final goodbyes, we left the hospital with Anna and Rachel. Anna was also being discharged that day, and Rachel was as emotional as I was. We'd spent five weeks together talking, crying, and commiserating, and I was going to miss her.

To cap off our beloved children's accomplishments, we took Alyssa's cue and drove to the famous "Rocky steps" located only a few miles from the hospital.

Cameras in hand, we watched as Anna and Devin ran to the top. As they reached the last step, they turned to face us with huge smiles on their faces, fists soaring up and down over their heads like Rocky had done long before they were born.

Rachel and I hugged, tears streaming down our faces. We knew it was possible, some would say inevitable, that our children would eventually suffer a reoccurrence. Right now, that didn't matter.

If Devin's CRPS returns, I feel confident he can fight it. Thanks to Dr. Sherry and the therapists at CHOP, he now possesses the skills, knowledge, and courage to desensitize and strengthen his leg at the first sign of trouble. He made it through these last two horrific years and ultimately through five grueling weeks. He knows that if he can rise above and conquer this painful neurological syndrome, he can fight any adversity life throws his way.

Chapter 13

One Year Later

I would like to tell you that we all lived happily ever after, but Devin's story isn't a fairy tale. Anyone who has been touched by this illness or has a child with a chronic disease knows it isn't this simple. Huge battles are won, celebrated - then often fought all over again.

*   *   *

After five weeks in Dr. Sherry's program, Devin returned to Traverse City on October 2, 2009, with a detailed home exercise program and a smile on his face. He'd missed the first month of his sophomore year of high school, but with the help of some flexible teachers and good friends, he managed the transition back to school with ease. Off all medications and in top physical shape, he no longer needed any accommodations whatsoever.

For the first time in two years, he could independently see, focus, learn, and study with no side effects from drugs, distractions from pain, or worries about the next person who might bump his leg. Although he still felt a small amount of burning pain down his right leg, it was expected to slowly diminish and disappear.

Devin quickly jumped back into regular activities with his friends. Within the first week of being home, he began playing tennis and hiking through the wooded hills of the frisbee golf course. Our son was back, and we started to believe this nightmare was truly behind us.

Nonetheless, I knew any number of problems could cause a setback, chief among them the flu. Flu season was upon us, and so was the new H1N1 virus, popularly known as swine flu. With vaccine quantities limited, I was frantic to get Devin immunized. Thanks to Dr. Sherry's counsel, I was all too aware that if Devin were to come down with the flu, his CRPS symptoms could flare.

By now, I was an expert at being resourceful. In early October, I finagled a seasonal flu vaccine for Devin. Unavailable to most people because of high demand and short supply, it was only being offered to seniors, hospital patients, and health care workers. After a fevered explanation and a bit of begging, I convinced our local senior center to allow Devin to join their ranks and be vaccinated along with them.

Securing a dose of the H1N1 vaccine wasn't so easy. As quickly as it arrived in our small town, it disappeared. Devin's school was supposed to have a vaccination day in mid-October and again later in the month, but it was cancelled both times because of short supply.

Then we heard about a special vaccination clinic at the mall for high-risk children the last Saturday in October. After standing in line with their father for three hours, both Devin and Taylor – our daughter because of her asthma – received the shot. I breathed a huge sigh of relief, but my thankfulness was premature.

Two days after receiving her vaccination, Taylor began to cough. Presuming it was a cold or small bug, I shrugged it off, but over the next few days she developed an extremely high temperature with severe body aches and a worsening cough. Her symptoms were classic and her pediatrician confirmed she had H1N1. In all likelihood, she was exposed shortly before or even after receiving her vaccine, since it takes many days to take full effect.

I crossed my fingers hopeful that Devin's vaccine would kick in before he caught the flu from his now very ill little sister, but one week later, he woke up extremely achy with a fever and cough.

My father quickly prescribed him the antiviral medicine used to combat the flu, but the symptoms had already taken hold. Devin's legs, arms, and whole body became increasingly achy. Two days into it, his CRPS pain, mild but still present, worsened.

Sander and I had a bad feeling, but we remained optimistic

in front of Devin. As the flu symptoms subsided, we told him, so should the CRPS pain. I hoped we were right, but inside I feared the worst.

The flu went away 10 days later along with the accompanying achiness, but the newly increased familiar burning pain of CRPS remained. It was tolerable, at around a 6 on the pain scale, and Devin quickly jumped into his exercise and desensitization program as he'd been instructed to do at CHOP if his pain returned.

Completely self-motivated, he ran two miles each day, performed each and every exercise he knew, and patted down and slapped his leg for further desensitization each night. He even upped the ante on a daily basis, as he'd learned to do in Philadelphia.

Meanwhile, in spite of the flu and missing four full weeks of school at the beginning of the year, he finished his first trimester in all honors and AP classes with a 4.0 grade point average.

As his second trimester began, despite the increase in his pain, he attended school each day and performed well. He was highly resolved to desensitize his leg fast, and I really believed he would. We just had to be patient, like in Philly.

Over winter break, he was well enough to downhill and cross country ski with us for the first time in two years, but toward the end of December, he came down with another bad virus. Yet another virus struck the first week of January.

Some research suggests CRPS is associated with problems with the immune system and may in fact be an autoimmune disorder, and Devin's present state certainly fit the bill. No one else in our family was getting sick, but his immune system seemed to be shot.

To our dismay, with each virus, his pain worsened. By mid January, he was losing the battle. No matter how hard he exercised, his pain continued to spiral. By the beginning of February, he was back at a 10 on the pain scale and once again became homebound and fully incapacitated.

I'd known a setback like this was possible, but for it to happen so soon was heartbreaking, and we were completely devastated!

*   *   *

With some reinforcement from Dr. Sherry and the team at CHOP, we braced ourselves for a difficult ride during the weeks ahead. Devin didn't want to go back to CHOP. Even in his current state of despair, he was convinced he could recreate the program at home and exercise hard enough on his own.

We agreed to this, but we insisted on hiring a trainer from a local health club to work with him and provide moral support. No matter how motivated he was, we felt he needed some outside encouragement in order to put himself through this kind of torture. Imagine asking yourself to use a wrench to slowly pull out one tooth at a time, without anesthesia. This is a realistic description of the type of self-inflicted pain Devin experienced when doing his exercises.

I provided Devin's new trainer with numerous articles and had long discussions with him about this rare pain disorder. I prepared him for what to expect and instructed him on how hard to push Devin through his pain during the challenging weeks ahead. Once this was accomplished, Devin began working with his new fitness coach at the gym two to three days a week. The rest of the time, Devin exercised independently at home.

It took twelve long, horrific weeks of brutal exercise, with no assistance from pain medications or medical marijuana, before Devin finally told us his pain was starting to go down.

To hear that his body was responding once again to this grueling desensitization program was the most precious gift Sander and I could have asked for, and to our joy, his pain decreased with each passing week. By the end of April, it was once again below a 4.

So what if he'd missed seven straight weeks of school this trimester and was flirting with failing all his classes? That Devin could lower his pain at home without the help and support of the therapists at CHOP was truly empowering. Likewise, our son was reassured for the second time that medications and procedures were unnecessary and that the most effective way to handle his CRPS was through desensitization and intense exercise. Having fought through it successfully two separate times, he was now absolutely certain he no longer needed to rely on anything but his own motivation and sheer will.

*   *   *

Just as we were beginning to breath again, knowing that Devin was finally comfortable and his pain was back under control, Sander and I were disheartened to learn that what we'd thought was just an annoying and temporary side effect from the ketamine was actually something much more serious.

Devin had been experiencing something called "flashbacks" for the past year, ever since the completion of his last ketamine infusion. Initially, these worrisome blips occurred about once a week and lasted anywhere from 10 to 30 seconds. They momentarily stopped Devin in his tracks with the same hallucinations and visual distortions he'd had when hooked up to ketamine in the intensive care unit.

It was just before our trip to Philadelphia when Devin experienced his first long flashback. His face drained of color and expression and he suddenly stopped communicating. He stared into space, looked dazed and out of it, and finally put his head down. When he emerged from this lengthy, seizure-like trance, he told us he'd been bombarded by bizarre visual hallucinations and felt extremely high.

During the ninth week of his new training regimen at the gym, incapacitated and devoted exclusively to exercising his way through the pain of his newly inflamed CRPS, Devin told us his flashbacks and visual distortions were worsening. He informed us they were coming quicker than before, sometimes multiple times a day, and they were more intense. Soon, he complained that he was experiencing them all the time, with no break between them. He told us he felt like he was hallucinating and high on ketamine 24/7.

At the time, Sander and I felt close to our breaking point. Getting Devin's pain back under control was our sole focus. Truthfully, his worsening flashbacks were more than we could handle, so we pushed this issue to the side.

However, once Devin's pain began to diminish that spring, the seriousness of the flashbacks became unmistakably evident. As Devin attempted to catch up on some of the class work he had missed during the numerous weeks of missed school, he found that his on-going hallucinations and visual perceptual changes made it difficult for him to read. Even when he could make out the words, he couldn't process them. Normally, our bright son could have caught up with ease, but nothing seemed to be going in, and when it did, he couldn't remember it for more than a minute or so.

I was reminded of the year before, when I'd tried to have him study for a history exam in the ICU while hooked up to ketamine. It had been like trying to teach a brick wall.

I could no longer deny the obvious. My deepest fear – that Devin's brain would be affected by the massive amounts of ketamine he'd been treated with the year before – had been realized.

* * *

We made contact with two of the leading physicians using ketamine routinely for CRPS and asked if they'd ever seen anything like this. Each told us they had not. Shockingly, they suggested that either protocol hadn't been followed properly at our hospital or that our son must be abusing other psychedelic drugs. They adamantly denied that his hallucinations had anything to do with the ketamine, and they had no interest in further investigating his symptoms.

Ignoring their ludicrous comments about Devin using other psychedelic drugs, I wondered how they could so easily dismiss such a serious potential side effect of a treatment they were providing to patients.

Using ketamine to treat pain was still relatively new, and comparatively few patients had received this treatment for CRPS. Even fewer individuals taking ketamine were adolescents, which meant Devin might well be the first documented case of someone his age developing this horrific side effect. Whether or not these physicians had seen such outcomes in their own practices or whether our hospital had administered Devin's treatment differently than theirs (our hospital and physician carefully followed a well-known protocol) wasn't the point. This important piece of information needed to be provided to doctors and consumers and further investigated.

I knew I had an obligation to pursue this further, so I conveyed Devin's story to the director of the Reflex Sympathetic Dystrophy Syndrome Association (RSDSA). He immediately e-mailed Devin's story to all the physicians and researchers worldwide routinely working with ketamine. As I'd hoped would be the case, this stimulated some conversation regarding the safety and efficacy of using ketamine, especially with adolescents.

* * *

My conscience clear at least in terms of communicating to others what had happened to Devin following ketamine use, I once again began spending countless hours online, intent on getting to the bottom of Devin's new problem.

I googled "ketamine," "persistent," "hallucinations," "flashbacks," combinations of these words, and every other word that came to mind. Soon, I discovered an illness that seemed to fit Devin's exact symptoms. Hallucinogen Persisting Perceptual Disorder, or HPPD, is an extremely rare disorder found in drug addicts who routinely use or have used hallucinogens like LSD, PCP, or ketamine.

HPPD typically begins, I read, with flashbacks. Over a year or two, they occur more and more frequently until the individual experiences persistent visual perceptual hallucinations and sometimes the genuine persistent feeling of being high. These hallucinations aren't psychotic in nature and involve no break from reality. Instead, they include a constant imagery of changing colors and shapes, bright lights, mirror imaging, moving images, trailing, visual imprints, halos, and often large amounts of peripheral visual garbage or particles.

I became stricken with grief, guilt, and despair when the same article noted that HPPD is a potentially permanent disorder of the brain. If Devin had this rare but potentially life-altering illness, it had been directly caused by the ketamine we'd treated him with over and over again.

Every article we read referenced one particular physician, Dr. Henry Abraham from Boston, Massachusetts, an addiction specialist on faculty at Tufts University. He'd not only researched, written, and published dozens of articles on HPPD, he'd even named the disorder.

Sander called him, and by the end of May, Devin and I were on the road again.

* * *

Dr. Abraham's first order of business was to have Devin undergo a three-hour long quantitative electroencephalographic procedure called the QEEG at the Children's Hospital of Boston so that he could assess any deficits going on within Devin's brain. Although it would be another week before we received the results, we eventually learned that the QEEG not only validated Devin's HPPD, it also suggested an auditory processing disorder, significant language and reading deficits, and possible encephalopathy, or brain damage.

That afternoon, after the QEEG procedure, we met with Dr. Abraham in his private office in a quaint New England town just outside of Boston. He was older and very kind, and Devin and I liked him instantly.

He had carefully reviewed Devin's history, including the results of the Wechsler Intelligence Test Devin had taken only days before. Our son's shockingly low score of 76 placed his current cognitive ability within the borderline range of intellectual functioning.

After learning that Devin's increasingly debilitating symptoms had caused him to drop out of all his classes for the last trimester of school, Dr. Abraham performed his own cognitive and visual examination. He hadn't yet received the QEEG results, but following his evaluation, confidently told us Devin had classic HPPD.

He told us he'd seen slow and complete recovery from HPPD in about half his patients with no assistance from any medicine.

He also talked to us about the other half of his patients, those who continued to experience HPPD symptoms for life. Some learned to live with their hallucinations and were productive and happy, finishing college and enjoying successful careers. Others had extreme difficulty with their symptoms and learned to adjust their lives accordingly.

Dr. Abraham looked Devin and me straight in the eyes and told us that Devin, at least for the time being, would have to change all of his goals.

A thick fog settled in my brain, making it difficult to concentrate. With each word that came from Dr. Abraham's mouth, I felt a dagger hitting my heart.

"He may not graduate high school on time, if at all."

"He certainly will not go off to college with his friends."

"He will not be able to continue his high school education in the same traditional fashion, and you will need to investigate either home school or special education."

I snapped out of it as Dr. Abraham told us we should try hard to remain optimistic. Devin was young with a plastic adolescent mind and we should look at this as a potentially temporary blip in time. The miracles of the mind were great, he emphasized. We should remain hopeful that Devin's symptoms would resolve, but to be aware this could take many years.

"Your best friend at the moment," he emphasized, "is time."

Uneasy, I asked, "Shouldn't I push Devin to work his brain to help retrain it, similar to what we did with his body in Philadelphia? Maybe if we continually challenge his brain, it will desensitize itself and return to full function. Certainly we shouldn't just sit back and wait?"

Dr. Abraham earnestly replied, "That is exactly what you *should* do. Let time take its course. I'm a strong advocate of 'use it or lose it,'" he reinforced, "but with Devin, this has to be done while working towards slow small changes."

Kindly, he insinuated that if we pushed Devin too much, he could become discouraged and give up completely. This simply wasn't the time to be the heroic mother.

Our appointment over, Devin and I sat speechless for a few moments before finally rising and thanking Dr. Abraham. He asked us to keep him posted and said he would be in touch when he received the report on Devin's QEEG. He shook my hand and gave Devin a warm hug, and we silently left his office.

Neither of us spoke for almost half an hour as we waited for our cab. Finally, with watery eyes, Devin asked, "Do you think I'll have to live like this for the rest of my life?"

Holding back tears and forcing a smile, I told him I didn't know.

*   *   *

Once home, Devin quickly chose to put aside the depressing reality of his situation and instead focus on his friends, the piano, and being a happy-go-lucky teen.

Maybe it was because his pain was under better control, or maybe it was because he was 16 years old. I don't know, but I was astonished at how easy it was for Devin to jump right back into life with a positive attitude.

I sure had a lot to learn from this young man.

*   *   *

Soon after our return from Boston, Devin received a wonderful and timely invitation to join Sander's partner at her summer home on the Mediterranean Ocean in Greece. Melpomeni is Greek, and she returns to her home and family each summer for six weeks.

This invitation wasn't entirely out of the blue. In the last few years, Devin and Melpo had developed quite a friendship. From yoga on Saturday mornings to enjoying delicious homemade Greek food to teaching Devin about her passion for tea and music, Melpo's influence on our son had been significant.

Devin was excited by the invitation, especially since he'd missed summer camp the past two summers, and Sander and I accepted the invitation with relief. This was a great way to take Devin's mind off the ominous situation at hand.

Our son's three-and-a-half-week trip to Greece with Melpo in late June revived him in many ways. He spent a short period of time in Athens where Melpo had a family apartment and the remainder of the time at the beach home she shared with her brother's family in a small village on the Bay of Corinth.

Every morning, he and Melpo jogged three miles and then swam in the Mediterranean. She taught him rudimentary Greek, and he learned about her culture by living among her family and friends. Together, they did yoga, cooked, swam multiple times a day, hiked up mountains, spent time with her brother Taso and his family, ate blocks of feta cheese with each delicious meal, saw ancient ruins, explored some of the Greek Isles, and relaxed in this unbelievable paradise.

All told, these were magical weeks: with his pain diminished, Devin temporarily stopped worrying about his education and had the time of his life.

Sander and I, too, had a much-needed respite from our intense worry about our son. We enjoyed some increasingly rare one-on-one time and took long walks together, and finally we began sleeping again.

We were startled awake one morning at 3:00 a.m. by the ringing of the phone. Instantly, we panicked. A call at this hour had to be an emergency.

It was Devin, but the news was extraordinary. He'd just gone for his usual three-mile run with Melpo and then jumped into the ocean for a swim. He'd felt a strange sensation and at first thought his legs had gone numb. After thinking about it, he'd realized the water was too warm. Confused, trying to figure out this strange sensation, he'd finally realized he wasn't numb at all. Instead, for the first time in almost three years, his legs were completely pain free.

"Mom, the pain was completely gone! It's still completely gone!" he exclaimed.

Chills ran up and down my spine and tears welled in my eyes as I listened to my son. After years of watching him suffer and traveling around the country searching for a solution, his pain was finally gone.

It is hard to put my emotions into words.

*   *   *

So here I sit, one year later, yearning only to bathe in the joy of seeing my son pain free for the first time in three years and instead grieving over the serious situation at hand, ironically caused by the aggressive treatments Devin received during our long journey to get him here.

Plain and simple, out of pure desperation to stop our son's pain, Sander and I made a tragic mistake. Now we struggle to come to terms with the pain and guilt of knowing the dangerous hallucinogen we gave our son over and over again has potentially altered his life forever.

As parents, our primary purpose is to protect and care for our children. Logically, I know everything we did was a desperate attempt to help alleviate Devin's intractable pain. I am cognizant that we had no way of knowing he had a rare genetic predisposition for HPPD or that ketamine would trigger this terrible disorder. But truthfully, all the logic in the world cannot help me come to terms with what has happened.

I am greatly saddened by what could have been for Devin. He was so close to having his life back. After three long years, he finally beat his pain! If only we hadn't given him ketamine...If only we'd found Dr. Sherry's program sooner...

If only we'd known then what we know now, Devin would be living the carefree, pain-free existence of an intelligent, fun-loving 16-year-old boy with an extremely bright future. I am certain this will haunt me the rest of my life, but having said this, I am trying my best to ignore the "what ifs" and instead move on and accept the fact that "What will be will be." No matter how much I question our past decisions or how sick I feel inside, it will not change the simple fact that Devin's path has been altered and that I have no control over what his future will hold.

It has taken me time and heavy reflection to see that what is important now is to focus on the present. For now, simply seeing a smile on Devin's face is all that matters. He is happy and pain free, and in spite of HPPD, he is bright and capable with loads of friends and interests. He is an exceptional young man with exceptional gifts, and deep within my soul, I sense that this will all work out for him somehow.

I have seen Devin's inner strength and unending resilience over and over again. If he was able to fight the constant, debilitating pain of CRPS and beat it after three horrific years, then certainly there is a chance he can beat this, too.

Holding onto this thought helps me remain hopeful that, in time, Devin's story may have a fairy tale ending after all.

Epilogue

Looking Back at Lessons Learned;
Looking Ahead with a Heartfelt Hope

As I sit back and reflect on this harrowing journey of ours, I am not going to lie and tell you I believe it happened for a reason and that it's all tolerable because good things have come from it.

In my opinion, things don't happen for a reason; they just happen. There is absolutely no good explanation for Devin or our family to have gone through this nightmare, and we definitely would have been better off if we hadn't. What purpose could there be for a 13-year-old to experience severe and constant pain causing him to be debilitated and basically homebound for three years? It has taken Devin and our family to a region of hell most people are fortunate to never have to visit.

Despite this depressing reality, this experience has reinforced many good qualities about our family. It brought out Devin's inner strength, courage, and true character under duress. Our son somehow remained optimistic through the worst of times. The occasional swear word aside, he demonstrated bottomless courage, sheer determination, and innate grace over and over again.

This experience also reinforced the strength of our family unit, which remained close and caring throughout this unpleasant period of time. It revealed the ease with which my husband and I worked together for the benefit of our child while maintaining a unified front, and it reminded me how fortunate I am to have Sander as my partner for life.

In addition to our peril with Devin, we were dealing with the daily stresses of raising two other children. Ethan was a teenager at the developmentally appropriate peak of his teenage rebellious years (as all parents of teenagers know, managing these tumultuous years could be a book in and of itself), while our daughter Taylor, a pre-teen, had to be kept happy and busy and veiled from the drama all around her.

This could have been a wrecking ball for our family. With this magnitude of stress day in and day out, it is easy to see how easily a marriage could fall apart, an older teen could take advantage of this convenient distraction in order to get away with murder, or a younger sister could feel lost and abandoned. The fact that Ethan and Taylor are thriving and Sander and I have not only survived but are closer than ever is something for which I am deeply grateful.

To our wonderment, Devin emerged from these three difficult years with a new level of maturity and a different view of the world around him. Suddenly, he had an appreciation for the vulnerability of his health. Unlike most kids his age, he no longer took for granted having a healthy and strong body.

He also recognized the importance of good friendships and the support and love of his family. He acknowledged the toll his illness took on the rest of the family, and he often commented on how much he appreciated our support and everything we did to help him.

Most importantly, he acquired perspective. Things that typically cause teens angst became meaningless to him. No longer was waking up early and going to school a drag, as most of his peers would attest. Instead, he described getting up and going to school as a pleasure. To put it simply, it was a delight to be anywhere pain free, even at school.

As we left Philadelphia, he actually confessed, "I can't wait to go back to school. It will feel so good to wake up each morning with virtually no pain, see my friends, and just sit in class all day and learn. I don't care how hard my schedule is. It will be a piece of cake compared to what I've been through these last five weeks!"

Like Devin, I too see the world with clearer eyes now. The typical stressors that come from being a mother and having high expectations for myself and my children no longer crowd my mind. I may have said it in the past and genuinely thought I believed it, but now I truly understand the meaning of the words when I say, "The health and happiness of my family is all that matters." I am happy for this illumination; I only wish it hadn't taken a horrendous experience to get me to this profound realization.

As elated as I am to have found Dr. Sherry's program, I confess I feel shaken to the core by our experience. It has left me with a deep and permanent scar, one that as a mother I will never be able to fully disguise, but it has taught me some profoundly important lessons, too.

*   *   *

The biggest lesson I learned was the importance of maintaining hope and remaining endlessly optimistic on the outside even when inside I felt as if all hope were lost.

When treatments fail over and over again, it becomes easy to wonder if anything will ever work. You wonder, "How much more can my child take?" and then "How much more can I take?"

Devin's doctor in California was the first physician to provide us with realistic hope. Although most literature will tell you there is no cure for CRPS, she expressed to us that, given Devin's age, we should be searching for a cure rather than settling for a palliative approach of any kind. Her belief in Devin helped us realize we couldn't stop until we found the answer.

Because of her, each time my husband and I discovered a new treatment approach or a new doctor, we were optimistic it would be the answer. We saw some treatments work to a degree and others fail completely, but we always let Devin know there was more out there and that we would keep searching. We talked about *when* he was better as if it were a certainty. We talked about the things he would do when this time came. Over and over, we told him, "We will never stop looking for an answer."

Although Devin's strength and determination came from within, I truly believe our confidence and optimism allowed him to remain hopeful and positive throughout this ordeal. If we, his parents, gave up, why wouldn't he?

I also learned firsthand the importance of becoming a strong and endless advocate when it comes to your child's education and health care. During the most challenging situations, when all I wanted to do was curl up in a ball and avoid the conflict ahead, I had to remember to trust my instincts. Because I was advocating for the most important cause of my life, the health and well-being of my child, I was able to set aside my otherwise typical concerns about what other people would think or how I would be perceived.

Unfortunately, I also learned the hard way that few physicians truly understand pain and that this basic misunderstanding causes some doctors to mistreat their patients. We were fortunate to work with some very special people as we searched for the answer to Devin's illness, but we also encountered too many physicians who couldn't see past their own noses. It didn't help that few doctors have experience or even basic knowledge about CRPS. As I was confronted with this situation over and over again, I became extremely disillusioned with the field of medicine.

Discussions about this with my general practitioner father introduced me to a useful term describing what happened to Devin: "cubby holing." When physicians "cubby hole" patients, he told me, they use gross generalizations to profile them.

A simple example: sometimes women with young children go to their doctor complaining of general fatigue. Because they fit the profile, they are cubby holed as "burned out stay-at-home-mothers."

Sometimes this is the case, but sometimes something else – a genuine health problem of some sort – is going on. Doctors who start with predetermined assumptions cannot make accurate diagnoses. When diagnostic tests are inconclusive, such physicians often jump to a psychogenic cause for the pain.

I saw firsthand how, when the diagnosis wasn't clear, instead of listening closely and making an appropriate referral, physicians swiftly placed Devin and me into a convenient category that allowed them to conclude that family or psychological issues were the cause of Devin's pain.

I also learned that, unlike adults who are wired to attach an emotional reaction to their pain, kids can often acknowledge pain and instinctively respond to it without becoming emotionally invested in it.

Jill Bolte Taylor describes this beautifully in her book *My Stroke of Insight*: "I am reminded of how courageous little children can be when they become extremely ill. Their parents may hook into the emotional circuitry of suffering and fear, while the child seems to be adapting to his illness without the same negative emotional drama."

Many physicians evaluated Devin as he smiled and pleasantly reported to them that his pain was at a 7 out of 10 on the pain scale. More than once, a doctor expressed to me that he didn't believe Devin, that his pain score wasn't possible.

"There is no possible way he can be experiencing this level of pain and still be smiling and talking with me," was a typical response.

The problem was that Devin actually could do this and in fact did it all the time! Even when he was in significant pain, he could often enjoy the company of his friends and have a pleasant conversation with adults. Most of the time, he simply didn't wallow in his pain, like many of us adults do, but this a hard concept for many physicians to embrace. In their opinion, high levels of pain are correlated with physical limitations as well as crying, screaming, grimacing, and sadness.

By contrast, I was easily hooked into the emotional circuitry of watching my son suffer day in and day out. While Devin tried to embrace the things that made him most happy and reverted to being a fun, goofy teenager whenever possible, I became further depressed and incapacitated each day by his worsening condition.

Regardless of its root cause, the assumption by some physicians that Devin's pain wasn't real caused extreme stress for our family and wasted a lot of time, energy, and money. If I hadn't eventually trusted my instincts and moved on to new physicians, Devin would have lost his confidence in our ability as parents to find the help he needed and he also would have wondered if we too were questioning the reality of his condition. It was imperative he knew we believed in him throughout this difficult time, even when educated professionals were telling us otherwise.

The lesson I learned was this: *you know your child better than any physician or health care worker who is just meeting him for the first time.* When you know something is wrong or it just doesn't feel right, question it. If the answers don't make sense, go to another doctor. Qualified physicians, pain programs, and organizations that specialize in CRPS exist, but it can take some real digging or even a stroke of luck to find them. It is still hard for us to accept that, despite our backgrounds and resources, it took us two years to locate the appropriate treatment for Devin.

What is even more unfortunate is that this is a typical experience for most patients with CRPS. For this reason, in the final section of this book, I have written a simple *Pediatric CRPS Family Resource Guide* in which I list the organizations, programs, and qualified physicians within the United States who treat CRPS with a brief explanation of each and what sort of philosophy guides their approach. Such an easy-to-read, comprehensive, and detailed list would have been a lifesaver during our journey and would have prevented us from feeling like the proverbial hamster on the wheel, going around and around but never gaining any ground.

Who would have guessed that Dr. Sherry of the Children's Hospital of Philadelphia who finally provided the proper treatment for Devin practiced literally just around the corner from the physician who consulted with us while Devin was in our local ICU receiving the controversial ketamine infusions? How could Dr. Sherry's name not be presented to us when this treatment failed prior to this same doctor encouraging us to send Devin to Germany for a ketamine coma?

In hindsight, it is clear that we could have avoided giving Devin ketamine altogether had we discovered Dr. Sherry's program sooner. Likewise, Devin would not be living with Hallucinogen Persisting Perceptual Disorder had a better coordinated medical model of care existed for children with CRPS. Hopefully, this book along with its resource guide will help other families find an easier and safer path to helping their child with this syndrome.

Although it is important to exhaust every treatment possibility, at this point in the game, I am obviously biased as to which approach patients with CRPS should try first. Of course I advocate a philosophy like Dr. Sherry's RND Program. It was the safest and most effective treatment we tried, and in my opinion should be the treatment of choice, not only for children with this disorder but for adults as well. Some rehabilitation programs do offer physical and occupational therapies for adults with CRPS, but none offer weeks of intense therapy six hours per day as is the case at CHOP.

Would adults be willing to put their lives on hold and endure the torture of a program like this? I really don't know, but I hope that in the future, treatment approaches like Dr. Sherry's will be looked at more closely for adults with CRPS.

Knowing what I know now, I strongly recommend leaving any medically invasive procedures and medications as a last resort. I just wish we'd been able to follow this advice. I wish we had more quickly and efficiently found the right treatment program for our son. Most of the treatments Devin received were highly invasive and medically aggressive, and some were controversial, dangerous, and as it turns out, came with serious consequences.

I must clarify that although we wish we'd discovered Dr. Sherry's program sooner, we are forever grateful to many of the doctors who cared for Devin. These skilled and extremely qualified physicians were using the latest research and the most up-to-date information they could find about CRPS. They went out on a limb trying to help Devin and were tremendously happy to hear that we finally found the answer for our son. Drs. Chagnon and Bruining in particular will always have a special place in our hearts, and we remain deeply grateful for their care.

*   *   *

I could not complete this portion of this book without addressing our family's experiences with medical marijuana. The legalization of marijuana in the state of Michigan has helped many people, including our son. From our perspective, the law was timely and helped us avoid a potentially dangerous situation with Devin regularly buying marijuana on his own to relieve his pain.

Nonetheless, I became deeply disheartened by the many inconsistencies within the law that made using medical marijuana an extremely difficult and uncomfortable experience for our family. Even with my shiny embossed card stating I was Devin's legal caregiver, I still felt like a common criminal. After all, I was forced to buy cannabis illegally from a willing caregiver or risk having Devin purchase it from drug dealers on the street.

I never understood why caregivers and patients weren't allowed to discuss purchasing cannabis in public or why compassion groups or physicians couldn't provide us with a list of caregivers or locations where we could purchase it like any other drug. I never understood why, if medical marijuana was legal, I was meeting strange men in dark alleys in order to secretly buy it for Devin.

As I learned from our trip to the medical marijuana clinic, the legalization of medical marijuana means this drug is getting into the hands of people who have no genuine medical need whatsoever, people whose only goal is to use it recreationally.

These problems could and should have been anticipated and addressed prior to the passage of the law in November of 2008. As time goes by, I can only hope that sound regulations will create a dignified and safe avenue for the legitimate use of medical marijuana by patients who need it.

*   *   *

One last thought occurred to me as I searched for closure to Devin's lengthy ordeal. This journey of ours from start to finish drained not only our family's wallet but also the health care system of an inordinate amount of money. Upon reflection and after conservative calculations, Devin's medical care over the last three years encompassed thousands of miles of travel from coast to coast and over $400,000 in medical costs. Although a portion of this came out of our own pocket, our insurance company was hit hard by Devin's highly misunderstood and rare condition.

Specifically, Devin endured assessments by 15 doctors, three hospitalizations, four weeks in two different intensive care units, 12 outpatient surgical procedures, an intrathecal spinal catheter, sympathetic blocks, lumbar blocks, a spinal cord stimulator trial, solumedral and bisphosphonate drips, a radiofrequency ablation, steroid and Botox injections, two week-long ketamine infusions, acupuncture, hypnotherapy, months of physical therapy, 14 failed medication trials, and 5 weeks in CHOP's RND Program.

Devin used to joke after each procedure that he had to sleep with one eye open since he was sure an insurance hit man was lurking beneath his bed to "take care of the problem." He would comically describe how he was just too costly and had to be discretely "taken out."

Literally hundreds of thousands of dollars in medical expenses could have been avoided if only more communication and a more coordinated medical model of care for this syndrome existed among physicians, and it is sad and a bit bewildering that this isn't the case. If we had been swiftly directed to Dr. Sherry's or another RND program, we could have avoided the majority of Devin's costly and unnecessary medical treatments and procedures, and Devin could have been spared a great deal of what he endured.

I suppose it is the complex nature of this disorder that has caused it to be placed under many different specialties of medicine, each with vastly different perspectives, but I would hate to see any other child or family go through what we have because of a communication glitch. This perplexing reality needs to be addressed, not only for the well-being of patients, but also for the health and well-being of our national health care system.

Above all, I hope this painful neurological condition will become better understood and better coordinated among health care professionals, with a more cohesive model of care and a clearer overview of treatment approaches, so that families everywhere can get the help they so desperately need early in their child's disease.

A Photo Collage – Devin's Journey

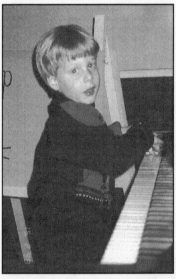

Devin playing piano at age three

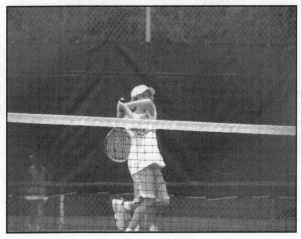

Devin, age 13, playing tennis before his injury

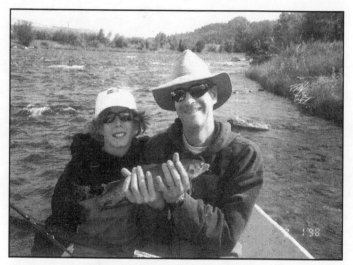

Devin and Sander at Yellowstone National Park before his injury

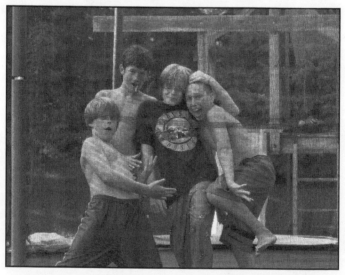

Devin (center) goofing off with his friends before his injury

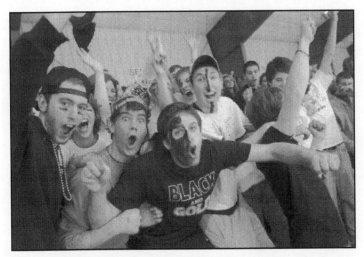

*Super fan Ethan at a Traverse City Central High School
basketball game his senior year of high school*

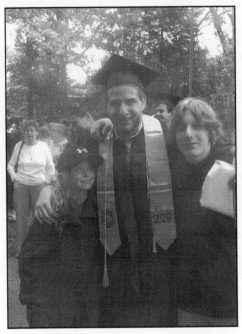

Devin and Taylor at Ethan's high school graduation

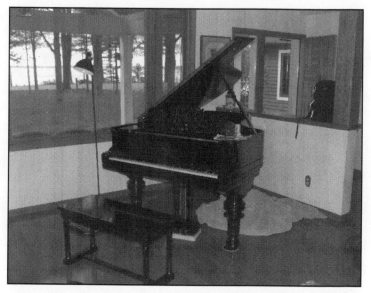

Devin's prize possession, his 1886 Steinway

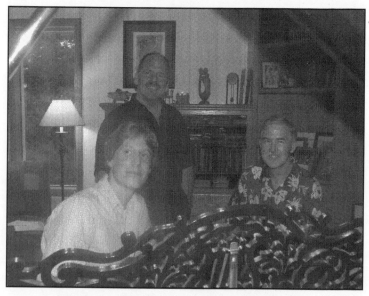

Devin after his piano recital with teachers
Jeff Haas and Michael Coonrod

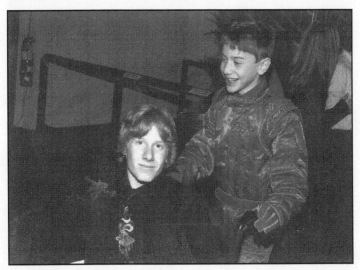

Devin being pushed in a wheelchair at his cousin's bar mitzvah

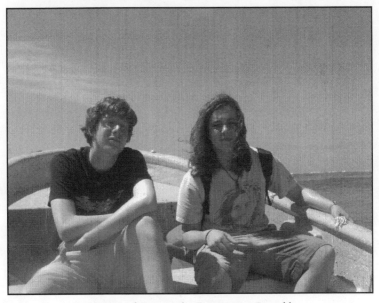

Devin and Eric in the Dominican Republic

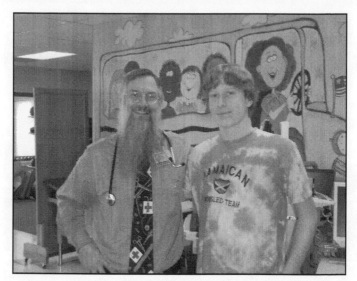

Dr. Sherry and Devin

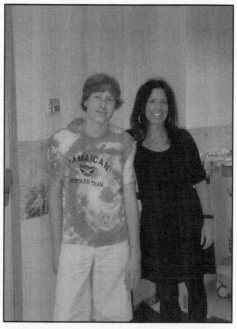

Devin and nurse practitioner Deb

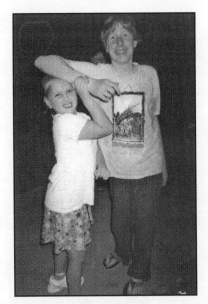

Devin and Anna

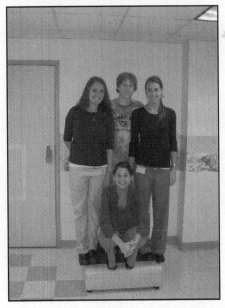

Devin with some of his therapists from CHOP

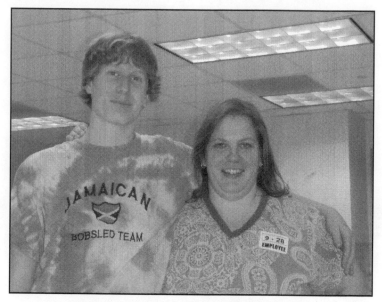

Devin with Lori, his physical therapy assistant

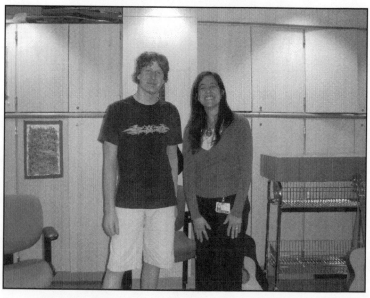

Devin with Amy, his music therapist

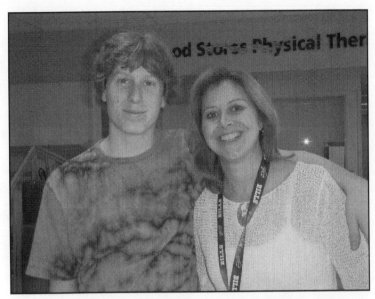

Devin with Tammy, his occupational therapist

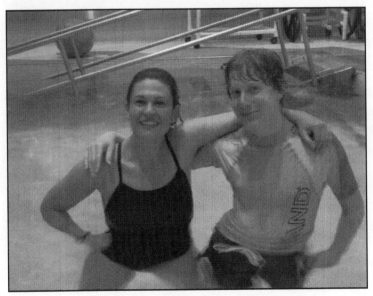

Devin with Tia, his pool therapist

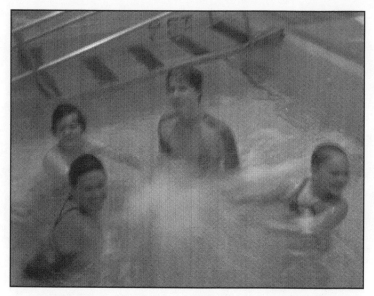

Devin in pool therapy

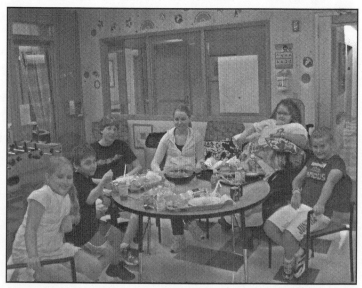

*Devin with fellow CHOP patients Anna, Morgan,
Benji, Mary, and Gillian during break time*

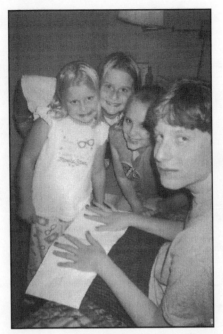

Devin getting his nails painted by the girls

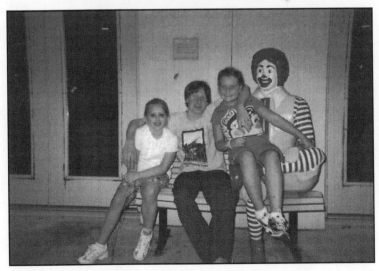

Devin, Anna, and Morgan sitting with Ronald

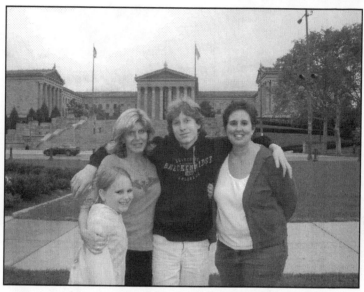

Devin and Anna with Rachel and me on their last day of the RND program right before they ran up the famous "Rocky" steps

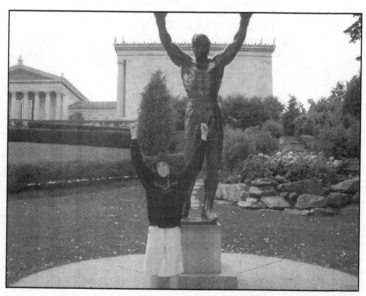

Devin in front of Rocky Balboa's statue

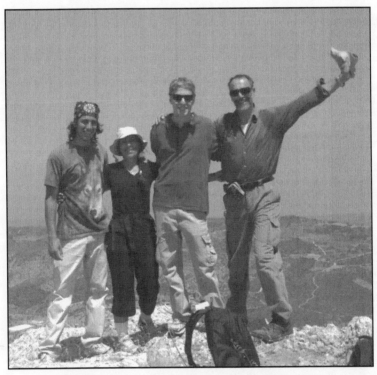

*Devin in Greece with Melpo, Taso, and Melpo's son
Chris on the top of a mountain overlooking the Bay of
Corinth with no pain for the first time in three years*

Pediatric CRPS Family Resource Guide*

Below is a summary of the different programs, physicians, philosophies, and organizations that treat Complex Regional Pain Syndrome. As we learned the hard way, many different worlds and conflicting philosophies exist. Although not exhaustive, the following guide should help you navigate the complicated world of pediatric CRPS and hopefully allow you to make the best possible choice for your child or adolescent. No matter which route you choose, make sure you are informed about each program's philosophy. Research each one carefully and only accept programs that are individualized to your child's needs. - Wendy Weckstein

(** Author's choice)

Reflex Neurovascular Dystrophy (RND) Programs**

These inpatient or day based programs work only with children and adolescents who have CRPS/RND. They are highly specialized and employ skilled therapists who are trained to work with this particular population. This approach is extremely effective and includes the use of physical therapy, occupational therapy, pool therapy, art therapy, music therapy, and psychology. Although overseen by a physician, it does not involve medical interventions or support from pharmacology. The program is individualized in length, typically between two and six weeks, based on the progress of each patient. The emphasis is on intense physical therapy, occupational therapy, and rigorous desensitization up to six hours per day. The intensity of the exercise, painful therapy, and absence of medical interventions is the crucial difference between this program and other interdisciplinary programs.

RND programs exclusively using Dr. Sherry's approach include the following:

Children's Hospital of Philadelphia (CHOP) Amplified Musculoskeletal Pain Syndrome Program
Dr. David Sherry, founder of the Childhood RND Educational Foundation

Legacy Emanuel Children's Hospital
Dr. Mark Shih
Based in Portland, Oregon, this program is modeled after Dr. Sherry's program.

Interdisciplinary Pediatric Pain Programs

These multidisciplinary programs are specifically designed to help children and adolescents with chronic pain caused by *various* diagnoses and are either inpatient or outpatient. Some are individualized in length while others are pre-set for a specific number of days or weeks. These pain programs use medical interventions and pharmacology to enhance progress if needed. Most interdisciplinary pediatric pain programs are customized to meet the specific needs of each child. Palliative pediatric pain programs, however, are less individualized. Here, many therapies are offered in a group setting. Counseling is a priority, with a large emphasis on teaching children coping skills and how to deal with their pain.

Specific interdisciplinary pediatric pain programs include the following:

The Mayo Family Pediatric Pain Rehabilitation Center (PPRC) at Children's Hospital of Boston at Waltham
Dr. Charles Berde, Medical Director
Dr. Navil Sethna, Clinical Director
This stand-alone partial day hospital provides intense outpatient programming for patients with chronic musculoskeletal and neuropathic pain, with Complex Regional Pain Syndrome the most common diagnosis referred to this center. This program combines intense physical therapy, occupational therapy, and cognitive behavioral therapy along with medical intervention from pediatric anesthesiologists, neurologists, and rheumatologists. This comprehensive program provides rehabilitation for children who have not responded to traditional outpatient therapy.

Cincinnati Children's Hospital Medical Center's Musculoskeletal Pain Clinic
Dr. Kenneth Goldschneider and Dr. Alexandra Szabova
The Cincinnati Children's Hospital Musculoskeletal Pain Clinic will evaluate children with CRPS and determine whether or not they require inpatient or outpatient services. The focus is on functional rehabilitation through physical and occupational therapy services after blocking pain through medication or other medical interventions if required. As inpatients, children receive three to five hours of physical and occupational therapy a day along with behavioral clinical psychology and other rehabilitation services as needed.

Cleveland Clinic Pediatric Pain Rehabilitation Program
Dr. Doug Henry, Medical Director
Gerald Banez Ph.D., Program Director
This pre-set three-week program involves two weeks as an inpatient and one week as an outpatient. Medical interventions and pharmacology are utilized as needed along with behavioral medicine. Other multidisciplinary treatments include psychology,

physical therapy, occupational therapy, recreational therapy, aquatic therapy, social work, and nursing care.

Connecticut Children's Medical Center Pain Relief Program

This program consists of three components, the Acute Pain Consultation Program, the Inpatient Pain Program, and the Chronic Pain Program. The inpatient program has a functional orientation and includes extensive physical and occupational therapy, psychology and educational support, and medical management. The typical stay is three weeks. The outpatient program consists of a multidisciplinary approach with the focus on regaining normal function. Recommendations often include medicine management, behavioral strategies, physical therapy, sleep counseling, and advice on school-related issues.

Duke Children's Hospital and Health Center Pain Evaluation Clinic

Dr. Laura Schanberg

The Duke Pediatric Pain Evaluation Clinic is dedicated to the assessment and management of pain in children. The physician-led team works together to assess each patient and includes a pediatric nurse, physical therapist, social worker, and psychologist. Their philosophy is to ease discomfort, maximize function, and promote full participation in daily activities. Following the evaluation, this multidisciplinary team will work with the child's primary care provider to help implement any recommendations.

The Blaustein Pain Center and the Kennedy Krieger Pain Management Clinic at Johns Hopkins

Dr. Sabine Kost-Byerly

At the Blaustein Pain Center, after an evaluation, the physician will provide interventional therapy such as neural blockades, spinal cord stimulation, and intrathecal therapy to inpatients. At the Kennedy Krieger Pain Management Clinic, the physician will assess the child and provide treatment in a multidisciplinary outpatient clinic. The child is evaluated by a physical therapist and a psychologist who specializes in pain management through behavioral medicine.

Lucile Packard Children's Hospital Pain Management Clinic at Stanford
Dr. Elliot Krane

This pediatric pain management clinic based in Palo Alto, California, provides individualized treatment plans to help inpatients or outpatients with various types of pain. The clinic uses conventional medical interventions and drug therapies as well as acupuncture, biofeedback, hypnosis, physical therapy, occupational therapy, and psychology.

UCLA Pediatric Pain Program at Mattel Children's Hospital
Dr. Lonnie Zeltzer

This pain program offers state-of-the-art medicine in combination with a multidisciplinary therapeutic approach and might include any number of the following holistic and more traditional therapies such as acupuncture, art therapy, biofeedback, energy-based therapy, hypnotherapy, massage therapy, craniosacral therapy, physical therapy, occupational therapy, yoga, individual psychotherapy, family therapy, school intervention, and/or medications. This individualized program offers both a traditional biomedical model of care as well as alternative, complimentary healing practices.

Mayo Clinic Pediatric Pain Rehabilitation Program
Dr. Tracy E. Harrison

Based in Rochester, Minnesota, this is a pre-set three-week outpatient rehabilitation program for adolescents with various types of chronic pain. The health professionals include physicians, psychologists, clinical nurse specialists, nurses, physical therapists, occupational therapists, recreational therapists, biofeedback therapists, pharmacists, dietitians, and education consultants. The program uses a behavioral therapy approach with the main emphasis on return to school, stress management, and parental involvement.

Nemours/Alfred I. DuPont Hospital for Children
Dr. Michael Alexander
This day hospital program based in Wilmington, Delaware, is designed for children with chronic pain, with the primary diagnosis being RSD or CRPS. It is individualized in length with four to six hours a day for two to five days per week. It involves intense physical therapy, occupational therapy, pool therapy, and psychological and academic services with the goal of increasing function, returning to school, and developing coping and management strategies. The goal is to decrease or eliminate medication if possible.

Rehabilitation Institute of Chicago Center for Pain Management Adolescent Pain Management Program
Dr. Norman Harden
This program provides an individualized approach for adolescents with various types of chronic pain involving occupational, physical, and cognitive behavioral therapies. Adolescents are seen two half days per week for up to eight weeks. The emphasis of this program is on exercise, relaxation, and coping strategies.

Ketamine Therapies

Currently, these are the most controversial yet highly successful pharmacologic treatments available. Rarely used with children, this treatment is considered extremely aggressive, somewhat risky, and highly invasive. Ketamine can be delivered orally as an inpatient five-day low-dose infusion (awake version), as an outpatient two-week low-dose infusion, or as a five-day ketamine coma, all with the goal of inhibiting the NMDA receptors and resetting the brain. The ketamine coma is only available at this time in Mexico and Germany.

Specific hospitals and physicians who supply ketamine treatment are as follows:

RSD/CRPS Treatment Center and Research Institute in Tampa, FL
Dr. Anthony Kirkpatrick

Here, research and clinical trials are currently being performed using a three-day high dose sub-anesthetic ketamine infusion. Participants receive this infusion as outpatients for four hours per day for three days. Dr. Kirkpatrick also evaluates and treats children with CRPS using therapies and medical interventions in the institute's state-of-the-art operating room. Dr. Kirkpatrick developed the International Research Foundation for RSD/CRPS.

Hahnemann University Hospital in Philadelphia, PA
Dr. Robert Schwartzman

Dr. Schwartzman evaluates and treats children with CRPS; he specializes in low-dose ketamine infusions followed by booster infusions.

Pain Clinics

Within these outpatient medical and surgical centers, physicians typically rely on pharmacologic or medical interventions to help lower the pain threshold so that functional rehabilitation through physical therapy is possible. These interventions may include sympathetic blocks, lumbar blocks, steroid injections, morphine pumps, spinal cord stimulators, radiofrequency ablations, and aggressive medication trials.

Holistic Medicine

Treatments that fall under this category include acupuncture, hypnotherapy, massage, biofeedback, nutrition, hyperbaric oxygen, and others.

Organizations/Websites

- **Reflex Sympathetic Dystrophy Syndrome Association, RSDSA** www.rsdsassociation.org
  Founded with the goal of promoting public and professional awareness of Complex Regional Pain Syndrome (CRPS), also known as Reflex Sympathetic Dystrophy (RSD), this website is designed to give patients, family members, and healthcare professionals information on the latest treatments and up-to-date legislation related to CRPS. It provides access to support groups, research, fundraising, and patient stories
- **American RSDHope**
  www.rsdhope.org
  This organization provides support, information, and education about Complex Regional Pain Syndrome to RSDS/CRPS patients, loved ones, friends, caretakers, medical professionals, and the general public.
- **Childhood RND Educational Foundation, Inc**
  www.childhoodrnd.org
  This non profit organization founded by Dr. David Sherry offers a website as a great resource where one can get videotapes, parent handout, links, and other material related to childhood reflex neurovascular dystrophy, RND
- **Mothers Against Chronic Pain**
  An organization of moms, dads, and concerned family members and friends that are looking for better ways to treat, cure, and take care of children who suffer from chronic pain conditions such as CRPS.

* List is not exhaustive. Programs and physicians are subject to change.

Acknowledgments

There are so many people I would like to thank for their help over the last two years. First, thank you to Ethan and Taylor for being understanding, patient, and independent, even when you would have preferred not to be, during all the time I was preoccupied and away. More importantly, thank you for being endlessly supportive, loving, and concerned about your brother throughout this lengthy period.

Thank you to Sander, my rock and my soul mate, without whom I would not have been able to survive this nightmare.

Thank you to my father, who remains one of the last old-fashioned family doctors. In spite of the limitations that come from insurance restrictions and the modern changes inflicted upon medicine, you continue to spend as much time as needed with each and every patient you see. You are one of the reasons I still have faith in the field of medicine.

Thank you to Dr. Michael Forness, Dr. Stephen Winston, Dr. Henry Abraham, Chris Parker M.S.W. and Lisa Zahn P.T. for your expertise and help along the way.

A very special thank you to Dr. Amy Chagnon and all the people at Sonoma Valley Hospital in California who cared for Devin when he spent 15 days in your ICU. Dr. Chagnon, your incredible amount of knowledge about CRPS gave us our first real hope that we could find a cure for Devin. Thank you for spending an inordinate amount of time providing him with quality care and the latest treatments available. Thank you for bringing exotic animals to the hospital just for Devin, even though he never had a chance to see them. Most importantly, thank you for believing in him.

Thank you to Dr. Kersti Bruining, a truly special person and doctor. We thoughtfully handpicked you as Devin's neurologist and primary physician in our hometown because you were one of the few doctors who listened to Devin and took the time to help us pursue proper treatment. Even though you weren't an expert in CRPS, you spent an unheard of number of hours researching and calling experts in the field so you could do everything humanly possible to help him. This included getting our local hospital to agree to allow you to administer a cutting edge, controversial treatment. Somehow, you even miraculously convinced our insurance company to pay for two ketamine inpatient infusions, which no one in the country had successfully done to date. In addition, thank you for offering your medical editing expertise along the way.

I also want to thank all the people in the ICU at Munson Medical Center in Traverse City, Michigan, for your skilled care and the personal time you spent with Devin and our family while he spent two weeks on your floor. In particular, thank you Dr. Robert Sprunk, Dr. Joseph Will, Dr. Richard Burke, and Dr. Terry Baumann for agreeing to be part of Devin's ketamine team.

I also want to thank all of Devin's friends for your endless and exuberant support. During the most difficult of times, you were the only ones who could bring a smile to his face. Thank you especially to Eric, Alex, Matt, Garrett, Keanen, Greg and Molly for sticking with Devin in the hallways at school when he could barely walk, even if it meant being late for lunch. Molly, thank you in particular for acting as Devin's mother hen, collecting his homework, studying with him, explaining to teachers what was going on when they didn't understand, and running with him almost every day when he returned home from CHOP.

Thank you to all of Devin's teachers at East Middle School and Central High School who have had to make the best of a rather difficult situation. Your flexibility and support have been greatly appreciated.

Thank you to Erin Kosch, Courtney Biggar and Bryan Burns, Devin's 504 coordinator, special education teacher and special education principal at Central High School, for providing Devin with different learning options and taking care of exceptionally challenging scheduling issues. Your support and creativity have kept Devin on track to complete high school with his peers. We are extremely grateful!

To Michael Coonrod and Jeff Haas, Devin's classical and jazz piano teachers, thank you for providing Devin with a respite from his pain and a medium through which he could express himself. Thank you for your patience when he could barely practice and your enthusiasm when he was able. You have become wonderful role models and very special people in his life.

Thank you to Melpo for your gift of friendship and for adopting Devin as your own. The time he spent with you and your family in Greece was truly magnificent.

To Becky Chown, my editor, thank you for sharing this extremely personal journey with me and helping me to clarify my thoughts when I was at my wit's end. I couldn't have done this without you.

Thank you to Rachel and Laurie for being my support system while in Philadelphia, and of course thank you to Dr. Sherry, Deb, Lori, Christie, Kate, Kira, Tammy, Tia, April, Amy, Kathy...I know you understand that it is hard to express my gratitude. You gave Devin his life back and ended our nightmare. Your program was the answer, and each and every one of you played a huge part in making it happen. *Thank you* from the bottom of our hearts.

Last but never least, thank you to Devin, with whom I spent thousands of hours over the last three years driving to doctors' appointments, sitting in hospital rooms, flying all across the country, sharing hotel rooms, and comforting, both at home and away. You have shown me the true meaning of determination and courage. You are my hero.

Thirty percent of all proceeds from *The Burning Truth* will be donated to:

The Reflex Sympathetic Dystrophy Syndrome Association (RSDSA) and,

The Childhood RND Educational Foundation

Made in the USA
Lexington, KY
05 October 2012